Haynes

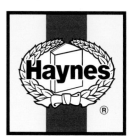

Baby
Manual

Including extracts from

Haynes Alcohol Awareness Manual by Gaylin Tudhope (ISBN 978 1 84425 295 4)

Haynes Brain Manual by Ian Banks (ISBN 978 1 84425 371 5)

Haynes Man Manual by Ian Banks (ISBN 978 1 84425 616 7)

Haynes Sex Manual by Ian Banks (ISBN 978 1 84425 086 8)

Haynes Teenager Manual by Dr Pat Spungin (ISBN 978 1 84425 409 5)

Haynes Woman Manual by Ian Banks (ISBN 978 1 84425 182 7)

Ian Banks

Cartoons by Jim Campbell

Haynes Publishing
Sparkford, Yeovil, Somerset BA22 7JJ, England

Haynes North America, Inc
861 Lawrence Drive, Newbury Park, California 91320, USA

Haynes Publishing Nordiska AB
Box 1504, 751 45 Uppsala, Sweden

British Library Cataloguing in Publication Data:
A catalogue record for this book is available from the British Library

ISBN: 978 1 84425 759 1

Printed in Britain by J. H. Haynes & Co. Ltd., Sparkford.

The Author and the Publisher have taken care to ensure that the advice given in this edition is current at the time of publication. The Reader is advised to read and understand the instructions and information material included with all medicines recommended, and to consider carefully the appropriateness of any treatments. The Author and the Publisher will have no liability for adverse results, inappropriate or excessive use of the remedies offered in this book or their level of effectiveness in individual cases. The Author and the Publisher do not intend that this book be used as a substitute for medical advice. Advice from a medical practitioner should always be sought for any symptom or illness.

Contents

Foreword

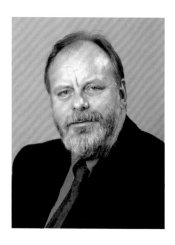

Given the paucity of baby books for dads we shouldn't have been surprised at the huge success of the Baby Manual first edition, but we were. All the plaudits said men would not be interested in a book on looking after offspring in their early dribbling years, let alone pregnancy or childbirth itself. Some hinted that this was *women's* business and showing full nappies and breastfeeding would simply turn men off. Well, the book sold in thousands showing that men as dads really *do* want to know how to cope with fatherhood. More to the point, men recognise that, through better understanding, the joy of being a dad far outweighs the worry and stress. So here is the second edition. It is bigger, better and, like a baby, learned from previous mistakes or omissions. Every comment sent in was taken into consideration. It's still directed primarily towards men as dads but many mums will find it useful as well. Although the information is reader-friendly we avoid patronising men; dads have their role to play and enjoy. There are brand-new sections, but the fun of having a baby, making sure they are safe, giving support for your partner and the iconic 'fault finding charts' are all still there and updated. So are the full nappies.

Author's acknowledgements

It is now a few years since the first Baby Manual appeared on the shelves of not only bookshops but also car spare-part stores. My thanks to the hundreds of people who took time to kindly comment not only on its value but also which areas were missing or could be better dealt with. People from organisations such as Sure Start, the Men's Health Forum, the Family Planning Association, NHS Direct and the British Medical Association, amongst many others, were indispensable. Alison Healey, Breastfeeding Coordinator Ashton, Leigh and Wigan PCT was so keen to see breastfeeding sufficiently highlighted she wrote the section. Material is also included from the following Haynes manuals: *Teenager* (Pat Spungin) and *Alcohol Awareness* (Gaylin Tudhope), *Brain*, *Man*, *Sex* and *Woman* (Ian Banks). Particular thanks to Ian Barnes and Simon Gregory for editing and factual checking. Jim Campbell's cartoons say everything while Matthew Minter made Baby Manual Edition II greater than the sum of the parts.

Dedication
This book is dedicated to my older sister Eileen Beaumont. But I'm still not fond of sprouts.

How to get the best from your GP

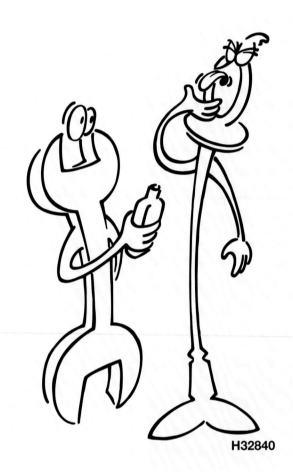

Do your homework with our insider information

Surgery telephone lines will be busier at certain times of the day and week. When you make an appointment ask your practice receptionist about the best times to call to cancel your appointment should you need to.

Write down the symptoms before you see your doctor
- It is easy to forget the most important things during the examination. Doctors home-in on important clues. When did it start? Did anyone else suffer as well? Did this ever happen before? What have you done about it so far? Is the baby on any medicines at present?

Arrive informed
- Check out the net for information before you go to the surgery. There are thousands of sites on health but many of them are of little real use. Click on NHS Direct as a start, or look in *Contacts* at the back of this book for up-to-date and accurate information.

Ask questions
- If a mechanic stuck his head into the bonnet of your car you would most certainly want to know what he intended. This doctor is about to lift the lid on your baby's body. Don't be afraid to ask questions about what a test will show, how a particular treatment works, and when you should come back.

Don't beat around the bush
- With an average of only seven minutes for each consultation it's important to get to the point.

Listen to what the doctor says
- If you don't understand, say so. It helps if they write down the important points. Most people pick up less than half of what their doctor has told them.

Have your prescription explained
- Make sure you know what it is for. Are there any side effects you should look out for?

If you want a second opinion say so
- Ask for a consultant appointment by all means but remember you are dealing with a person with feelings and not a computer. Compliment him for his attention first but then explain your deep anxiety.

Flattery will get you anywhere
- Praise is thin on the ground these days. An acknowledgment of a good effort, even if not successful, will be remembered.

Be courteous with all the staff
- Receptionists are not dragons trying to prevent you seeing a doctor. Practice nurses increasingly influence your treatment. General practice is a team effort and you will get the best out of it by treating all its members with respect.

H32840

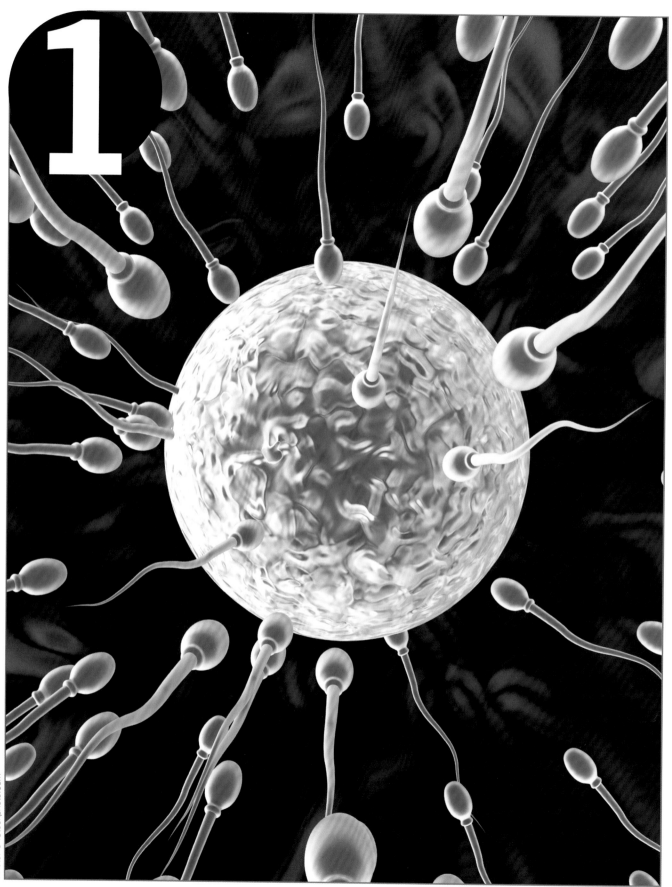

1

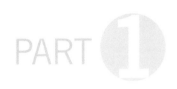

PART **1**

BABY MANUAL

When and how to conceive

PART ① **Contraception**

Introduction

There are numerous methods of contraception, most of which, it has to be said, depend more on the woman than the man. Not only is there a difference in the way the methods work and are used, but there is a significant difference in the protection each method provides.

The male condom

Society is increasingly accepting the condom as one of the normal requirements of modern life. This has led to their wider availability and condoms can now readily be obtained – in supermarkets, from garages, by mail order, through slot machines, as well as in pharmacies. They are free from all family planning clinics and genito-urinary medicine clinics. Colours, flavours and new materials, like plastic, make interesting options. Condoms now come in different shapes and sizes, and it is often necessary to try a few different types before the right one is found. If used correctly condoms are 98 per cent effective at preventing pregnancy and they have the added advantage of providing good protection against many sexually transmitted infections. Hermetically sealed, the modern condom will remain usable for a long time (look for the expiry date); good quality condoms will also have the CE mark and the kitemark. Once the seal is broken they should be used quite soon as the rubber will perish on exposure to the air and the lubricant will dry, making it difficult to put on.

Use of condoms

Using a condom correctly is essential for it to be effective. It should be put on before any contact between the penis and the vagina or genital area, and rolled on the correct way round. Air should be excluded from the end of the condom as it can cause

Can you re-use a condom by turning it inside out?

Desperation is truly a terrible thing. The short answer to this question is yes, but your choice of sexual acquaintances may be severely restricted afterwards. You could also be a daddy as sperm can survive for a short space of time in the air. Additionally you may also contract just about any sexually transmitted disease going. But yes, you can re-use a condom by turning it inside out just like you can wear three day old socks by the same manoeuvre. On the other hand, it is probably best to shell out for another packet or have a cold shower. Both are a good deal cheaper in the long run. If you plan ahead, you can get them free from the Family Planning Association.

Can you get pregnant while you are breast-feeding?

This question is usually asked by the father of twelve children. Although there may be a prolonged delay in the resumption of periods, and thus ovulation, there is no way of knowing just when it is going to start. Obviously an egg has to be released for a period to follow. If unprotected intercourse takes place at this time there will be an even more prolonged delay. Getting pregnant is another excellent way of stopping periods.

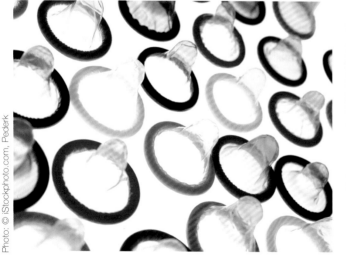

Photo: © iStockphoto.com, Pederk

The condom

Is butter or margarine a good lubricant when using a condom?

No to both, even if you would never know it wasn't butter. Oil-based lubricants dissolve latex condoms. Butter, margarine, cooking oil or even WD40 will produce a slippery slope towards a drippy willy not to mention unwanted fatherhood. Use only water-based lubricants.

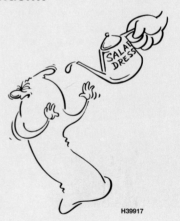

H39917

it to burst or slip off. Sharp finger nails, rings and teeth are a hazard. Only the soft finger pulps should be used to unroll the condom on to the penis. If extra lubrication is needed then only a water based one should be used with rubber condoms. There is a need to withdraw and remove the condom while the penis is still erect to avoid semen leaking out as the penis shrinks in size.

Spontaneity
Perhaps the single biggest stated reason for not using condoms is the widely held belief that they inhibit spontaneous sex. Foreplay is an important part of enjoyable sexual activity and partners can involve the condom in this. Fears that they reduce the sensitivity of sexual experience have not been supported by research. Most of the problem is with the psychological inhibition some men have over their use but without doubt lots of foreplay does help.

The female condom
The condom for women is relatively new, but regular users report favourably and many men prefer them to the male condom. Made of plastic it is larger in diameter than the male condom and has a flexible ring at each end. The smaller ring fits inside the vagina while the outer, larger, ring remains on the outside of the vagina. After ejaculation this outer ring should be twisted to prevent escape of the sperm and the condom gently withdrawn. Female condoms are 95 per cent effective, and also have the advantage of providing protection against many sexually transmitted infections.

Oral contraception (the Pill)
The combined pill contains two hormones which inhibit the release of the hormones which stimulate the final development and release of ova (eggs) from the ovary. This partly mimics a pregnancy, which explains why some women suffer the milder symptoms of being pregnant when using this pill.

The combined pill is convenient, over 99 per cent effective when taken correctly, and has many advantages (including protection against cancer of the womb and the ovary). Like all drugs, there are health risks associated with its use. A very small number of women will develop a blood clot which can be life-threatening. Women who take the pill are also more at risk of being diagnosed with breast cancer or cervical cancer. However, for the vast majority of women the advantages of taking the pill greatly outweigh the risks.

The progestogen-only pill contains only one hormone and stops sperm from getting anywhere near the egg by maintaining the natural plug of mucus in the neck of the womb. It also makes the lining of the womb thinner. It is highly effective (99 per cent) and it is particularly useful for women who cannot use

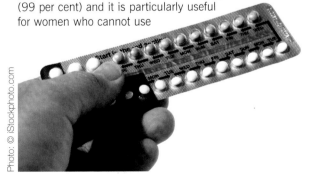

Photo: © iStockphoto.com

The Pill

the combined pill, and those who are breastfeeding. It has, however, to be taken regularly at the same time each day, and can have the disadvantage of causing irregular bleeding.

Intrauterine contraceptive device (IUD)
These small plastic and copper devices are inserted into the womb by GPs, or by doctors or nurses at family planning clinics. They prevent pregnancy by stopping the sperm and egg meeting; they also make the lining of the womb unsuitable for implantation should fertilisation occur. They are over 99 per cent effective, can be left in place for up to eight years, and can be used by women both before and after having children. They are not suitable for women who are at risk of getting a sexually transmitted infection, and can make periods longer and heavier. To minimise the risk of infection, tests are done before the IUD is put in. The IUD is removed very easily by a doctor or nurse and has no effect upon sensation during intercourse.

Intrauterine contraceptive system (IUS)
These small plastic T-shaped devices contain the hormone progestogen. They are inserted into the womb by GPs, or by doctors or nurses at family planning clinics. They prevent pregnancy in the same way as the progestogen-only pill. They are over 99 per cent effective, can be left in place for up to five years, and can be used by women both before and after having children. Initial side-effects can include irregular bleeding, but periods then tend to become lighter and shorter, or stop altogether; period pain is also reduced. Like the IUD, the IUS is removed very easily by a doctor or nurse and has no effect upon sensation during intercourse.

Hormone implant (for women)
One small rod containing progestogen is inserted under the skin in the arm, usually using a local anaesthetic. It works like

How long after sex can you take the morning after pill?

The so-called emergency contraceptive pill is simply a very high dose of sex hormones. It prevents a fertilised egg from implanting on the uterine wall. One dose is taken immediately followed 12 hours later by another. After 48 hours the chances of preventing pregnancy begin to decline. If left too long there is a theoretical danger of damaging the developing foetus without stopping the pregnancy. You will need a pregnancy test performed three weeks afterwards.

It is very effective but not in the same league as the oral contraceptive pill itself. You need a doctor's advice if you suffer from high blood pressure or have ever had a problem with blood clots.

the progestogen-only pill and lasts for three years. The main disadvantage is that it can cause irregular bleeding for several months. It is over 99 per cent effective and is easily removed in a minute or two.

Hormone injection (for women)

The hormone progestogen is given as an injection every 8 or 12 weeks, depending on the type used. It is over 99 per cent effective and works by stopping the ovaries producing eggs. It shares many of the advantages of the combined pill, but can cause irregular bleeding and weight gain. Once the injections stop it can take a year or more for periods to return.

Contraceptive patch (for women)

This is a small patch, like a sticking plaster, which is applied to the skin to protect against pregnancy. It releases two hormones into the bloodstream and, like the combined pill, stops the ovaries releasing eggs. It also thickens the mucus around the cervix, making it difficult for sperm to get into the womb. Each patch is worn for seven days, and after the third patch none is worn for a week, when some bleeding may occur. At the end of that week the 21 days-7 days cycle starts again. It is important to change the patch on the correct day, and apply a new one immediately if any fall off.

The effectiveness and side-effects are as for the combined pill, and may also cause headaches and skin problems. It does not protect against sexually transmitted infections.

The male Pill

The day when a male pill will be available slowly gets nearer. There have been successful human trials in the UK, and in the next decade we should see a male hormonal method of contraception. At the moment it is unclear whether this will be in the form of a pill, an implant or an injection.

Female sterilisation

This is a permanent method of contraception in which the fallopian tubes are either cut, sealed or blocked so that eggs cannot pass down them to the uterus (womb). It has a failure rate of 1 in 200, making it 99.5 per cent effective – as good as other long-term reversible methods. Should it fail, it carries a greater risk of the egg implanting in the fallopian tube (ectopic pregnancy). As a

general anaesthetic is required and the operation is more invasive it is a more complicated and risky procedure than vasectomy. It is possible to reverse the operation but with limited success, and with an increased risk of ectopic pregnancy.

Emergency contraception

'Emergency' contraception is a safe and effective way of preventing pregnancy. It involves either taking tablets containing progestogen (which are used within 72 hours of sex but are more effective the sooner they are taken) or inserting an IUD. Emergency methods can be used when no contraception was used or when regular contraception has failed. Emergency pills are safe to take and have no lasting effects on future fertility. Emergency contraception is available free from GPs and family planning clinics. In addition, emergency pills are free from NHS Walk-in centres and can be bought from pharmacies by women over 16.

Does masturbation make you deaf?

Given the horrendous hours junior doctors work, asking any casualty officer this question will invariably prompt a reply of 'Pardon?' In truth masturbation doesn't affect your hearing. Worse still it has no such effect on your mother's hearing either, who invariably rushed into your bedroom thinking you were being attacked by a Doberman with a stutter. Woody Allen knows a good thing when he experiences it. 'Don't knock it' he said in the film *Annie Hall*, 'it's sex with someone you love'. The Talmud states categorically, 'Thou shalt not masturbate either with hand or foot'. Yes, masturbation may not make you deaf but catching a genital verucca off your own foot really is the pits.

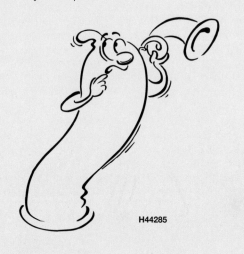

H44285

Is petroleum jelly the best lubricant?

Yes, is the answer if you are talking about a baby's bum, but for use with a condom you would be wiser using sandpaper. At least you would feel the condom falling to pieces. Petroleum based lubricants will dissolve most condoms, particularly the ultra-thin varieties. Always use water-based lubricants; they are also a less of a fire risk during burning passion.

Can you use a tampon to prevent pregnancy?

There is a doctor in England who uses tampons to stop severe nose bleeds. Walking around with a tampon up your nose has not yet hit the television advertisements. I suspect you might not feel quite so free if you walked into the local transport cafe in this nasally disadvantaged state. Tampons are a marvellous invention for soaking up blood such as the menses, or a nose bleed for that matter. Unfortunately they are not quite so good at stopping little genetic torpedoes hell bent on being the first successful headbanger. Not only will they not prevent pregnancy, they have even less protection against sexually transmitted diseases.

Part of a casualty officer's life is taken up by removing these items after being rammed home in a fashion not unlike loading a cannon. Worse still they can be forgotten and fresh tampons used for the rest of the period. Removing them can then be hazardous as the tampon becomes saturated with offensive bugs a lot worse than headbangers. Septic shock is no joke and lives have been lost, so de-tampon before the fun with your ramrod, if you follow my drift.

Natural methods

It is only possible for your partner to conceive within 24 hours of ovulation. However, because sperm can live for several days, sex that happens up to seven days before ovulation can result in pregnancy (this sex can even be during a period). It is possible to estimate the fertile period by noting certain changes in the body. Using a fertility thermometer and a chart it is possible to detect the sudden rise in temperature of around 0.2 degrees Celsius which occurs at ovulation. Monitoring changes in the cervical mucus help identify the time before and after ovulation. The mucus becomes thin, watery and clearer before ovulation, and

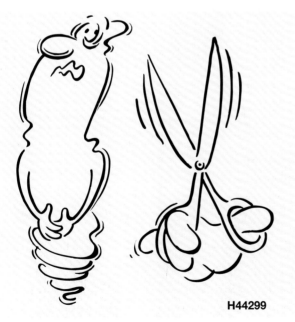

H44299

Vasectomy

afterwards returns to being thicker, stickier and whiter. When practised according to instruction, natural family planning is 98 per cent effective, although it does take a while to learn it as a method and requires commitment from both partners.

Vasectomy (male sterilisation)

Vasectomy is a simple and permanent method of contraception. You don't need permission from your partner but obviously it makes good sense. Fortunately there is no reported effect on enjoying sex. The testicles continue to produce sperm but rather than being ejaculated with the semen the sperm are reabsorbed in each testicle. Sperm therefore doesn't build up inside the testicles. As with any surgical procedure you will have to sign a consent form.

When it should be done
Although there is no lower age limit for vasectomy, young, childless men need to consider this method carefully to avoid later regret. It should therefore only be chosen by men who, for whatever reason, are sure that they do not want children in the future. Counselling is recommended so that other contraception options can be discussed and the procedure fully understood. A vasectomy immediately following a birth, miscarriage, abortion or family or relationship crisis is a usually a bad idea.

How it is performed
You can ask for a general anaesthetic but it is generally performed under a local anaesthetic. A small section of each vas deferens – the tubes carrying the sperm from the testes – is removed through small cuts on either side of the scrotum. The ends of the tubes are then cut or blocked. Stitches are rarely required on the scrotum. It is a simple and safe operation lasting around 10-15 minutes, and can be done in a clinic, hospital outpatient department or doctor's surgery.

Recovery
Discomfort and swelling lasting for a few days is normal but this settles quickly with no other problems. Simple pain-killers help. Occasionally this can last longer and needs your doctor's attention. Strenuous activity should be avoided for a week but you can return to work immediately and have sex as soon as it is comfortable. As the testicles continue to produce testosterone your feelings, sex drive, ability to have an erection and climax won't be affected. Despite numerous scares in the popular media, there are no known long-term risks from a vasectomy.

Effectiveness
After a vasectomy it can take a few months for all the sperm to disappear from your semen. You need to use another method of contraception until you have had two consecutive semen tests which show that you have no sperm. While vasectomy is highly effective failures are still possible (1 in 2000). The failure rate should be discussed before the operation and it should be pointed out on the consent form. While vasectomy is excellent in preventing pregnancy it will not protect against sexually-transmitted infections. Using a condom is the best protection for this.

Future prospects
Reversal operations are possible but not always successful and will depend upon how and when the vasectomy was done. Reversals are not easily available either privately or on the NHS.

PART **1**

Bloke's guide to pregnancy

Us men hate to ask for help but things could be better for everyone if we devoted as much time to understanding the mysteries of pregnancy as we do to understanding the conundrum of how the toilet seat is always down again next time we go to the bathroom.

Men are under increasing pressure to be more empathic during pregnancy and labour. Even Bill Crosby realised the

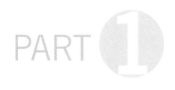

A baby is not a fashion accessory; don't do it until you're ready.

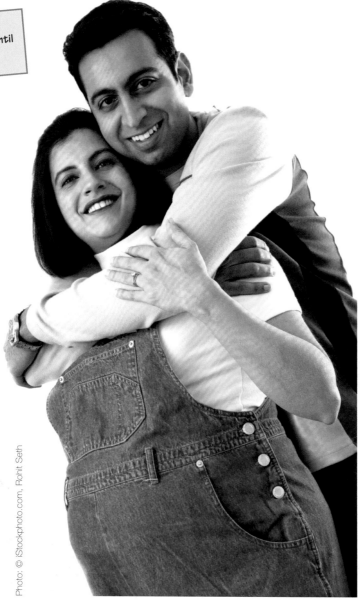

Photo: © iStockphoto.com, Rohit Seth

importance of seeing things from the woman's perspective. When asked was labour painful he answered, 'It sure is. She damn near squeezed the fingers right off me'. In truth, it is a joint decision between partners just how much the man should get involved. But a bit more insight makes the decision more informed and less of a knee jerk reaction.

Having a baby is more exciting than your team winning (honest)

Not all men are ecstatic on hearing the good news and there are invariably mixed emotions. Tearing all your hair out and ripping up your season ticket to Manchester United will not go down well. A bottle of champagne (of which you will be able to drink the greater part quite legitimately) most definitely will in all senses of the word.

Your partner will be offered a choice of ways in which she can have antenatal care. This will be influenced by her previous pregnancies, medical health and social factors such as living in a remote part of the country which only the flying doctor can get to in a rush. No matter what anyone tells you, being pregnant is not an illness and having babies may occasionally be a tad tricky but it is still normal and women have been doing it for a very long time. Women in their first pregnancy where there is some reason to want closer observation, or if a previous pregnancy was difficult, are often advised full hospital care. A named consultant and a named midwife will take responsibility for your partner's checks as she approaches her delivery dates. Parental classes are usually held in the same department, which is just great for ensuring as few men attend as possible. Pity, as they are great fun especially for us fat dads who empathise so much better. You are welcome to come along to these antenatal sessions, especially for the first ultrasound scan. Never underestimate how scared your partner can be at that first session. A hot sweaty hand in her hotter sweatier hand helps more than you will know. It's easy to forget in that darkened room with the glowing, totally incomprehensible screen that abnormalities are rare and all unusual positions in the womb can be safely dealt with.

Most GPs will offer a mix of checks at their surgery along with visits to the maternity hospital. Convenient and quick, it also ensures contact with a doctor who generally knows a lot about your partner's medical history. You can also attend these just like the hospital sessions. However, I have yet to find men beating a path to my door which is not surprising as most will only attend the surgery when they are in the terminal stages of a condition or Liverpool FC are playing Manchester United mid-week.

Early days, happy returns

Morning sickness baffles most men. Chundering after 10 pints and a curry is perfectly reasonable behaviour but to wake up with pursed lips and wide expectant eyes is patently odd. This can be so bad, especially in the first two semesters (6 months) women sometimes dehydrate, lose weight and need to be admitted to hospital. There is probably nothing you can do when it gets this bad but for the less traumatic versions many women find tricks to reduce the sickness. A small dry biscuit with a cup of tea or milk is a common strategy but it only works if it is there *when she first awakes*. Five minutes too late and your pillow has a permanent stilton flavour.

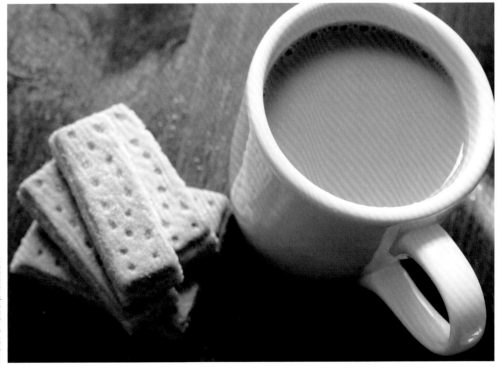

Photo: © iStockphoto.com

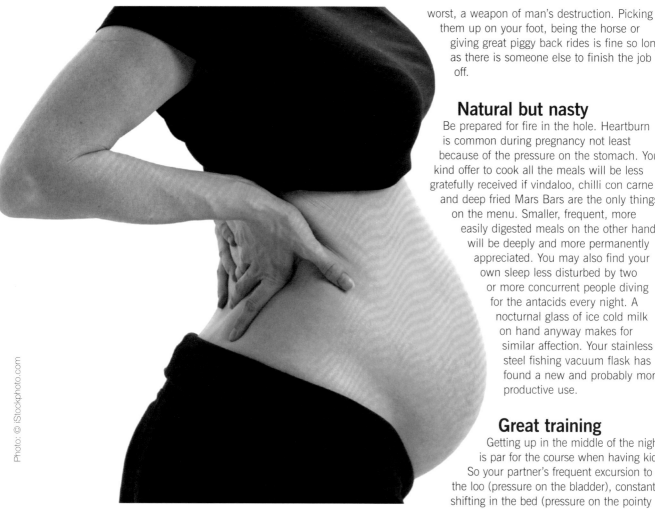

Photo: © iStockphoto.com

worst, a weapon of man's destruction. Picking them up on your foot, being the horse or giving great piggy back rides is fine so long as there is someone else to finish the job off.

Natural but nasty

Be prepared for fire in the hole. Heartburn is common during pregnancy not least because of the pressure on the stomach. Your kind offer to cook all the meals will be less gratefully received if vindaloo, chilli con carne and deep fried Mars Bars are the only things on the menu. Smaller, frequent, more easily digested meals on the other hand will be deeply and more permanently appreciated. You may also find your own sleep less disturbed by two or more concurrent people diving for the antacids every night. A nocturnal glass of ice cold milk on hand anyway makes for similar affection. Your stainless steel fishing vacuum flask has found a new and probably more productive use.

Great training

Getting up in the middle of the night is par for the course when having kids. So your partner's frequent excursion to the loo (pressure on the bladder), constant shifting in the bed (pressure on the pointy bits) and irrational demands for a life-saving Belgian chocolate at 3 am (hormone shifts) should be seen as great training. Leave the light on in the loo, buy a better mattress, give great massage and work out the shortest route to the all-night delicatessen. Toughens you up, boy, for the big push to come later. Sudden, swift and severe shifts in mood are also part of the equation as hormones leap around like demented jugglers. Expect weeping followed by ecstatic laughter at banal baby-product adverts. Join in. Has to be better than a party political broadcast. Now is the time for being Nelson Mandela not George Bush. Just because she can't explain why the bedroom has to be painted pink, the baby cot erected from a flat pack, the stairs cordoned off like East Berlin at 1 am *six months before the baby is even due* is perfectly reasonable to her. Think of it this way, if a man says something in a forest and no woman hears him say it, is he still wrong? Exactly.

You are going to have an interesting nine months with a finale that throws the Cup Final into a cocked hat *and* you will be on the winning side. Good luck dad.

Two to tango

When it comes to making babies Aristotle had a theory. The woman provided the canvas while the man supplied the paint. This is a pretty good reflection of male dominance in the medical profession. Housework can be a bit like that too. Supplying the canvas can be pretty hard work, not least because your weight is steadily increasing, pressure is building up on your diaphragm, bladder and digestive system and most importantly, your hormones are doing a samba with your emotions.

Being heavier is not just the problem, it's being heavier just in one place, the front. This puts strain on the back muscles so bending over or simply standing up straight, gets increasingly difficult. Watching out for when she has something to pick up and darting in like Sir Walter Raleigh, giving a back massage during the day as well as at night and more to the point, doing the housework all make for better tangos, if not sambas. You and I know that constant childcare is at best challenging and, at

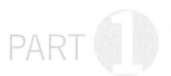

PART 1 **Timing is everything**

Introduction

Choosing the time of being a dad may not always be in your control, but if it is, there are advantages and disadvantages for young dad versus old dad.

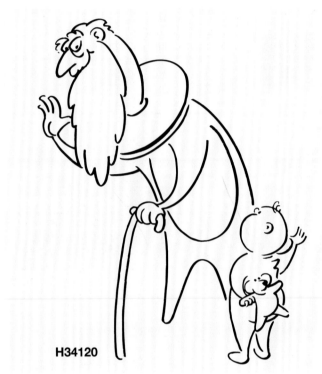

H34120

The older dad

Can semen give you cancer?

There is no evidence that semen causes cancer. From an evolutionary point of view, it wouldn't really make much sense if all the females of a species promptly died a horrible death every time they tried to procreate. A sort of 'go forth and divide'. For many years a battle ranged over whether sex with uncircumcised men caused cervical cancer. It was noted that virgin women never contracted cervical cancer and that Jewish women in Israel had a lower incidence than women in, say, the UK. Obviously, the scientists thought, it's all down to the foreskin. When all the statistics are examined more fully it appears that promiscuity is a greater factor and that the presence or absence of the foreskin is of relatively little consequence.

It is worth noting that one organism suspected of causing cervical cancer is Human Papilloma Virus (HPV). This is transmitted by unprotected sex with a carrier of the virus; as ever, condoms provide more or less total protection.

Teenage dad

Becoming a parent in your teens is generally best avoided if possible. Research shows that teenage mothers are significantly disadvantaged with regard to their standard of living later in life; teenage dads probably aren't much better off.

Young dad

You are going to need all the youth you can muster, especially in the first few weeks when the jet lag from the lack of sleep starts to kick in. On the other hand you will be able to take part in their games as they get older without snapping your Achilles tendon and be young enough to enjoy regained independence once they leave home. You are also less likely to employ a crowbar to lever the remaining son out of the family home. Before you shout 'brace yourself darling' just a word in your ear. You may be losing the best years of your life. Along comes responsibility, a whole new look at car maintenance for necessity not fun, lost mates, especially the car maintenance variety, financial commitments when your earning power is at its lowest and of course that haunting fragrance of damp nappy.

Middle-aged dad

It's easy to see the advantages of kids while you are in your thirties with more earning power, a good taste of the free unfettered youth, and your parents still around to do all the baby sitting while you swan off to breakaway holidays in the Antipodes but wait a second, mate. Work pressure is at its highest during your middle age especially with jobs under pressure from women. The life-long post is no more. Keeping on track with your career might be difficult with a few kids in the equation. Paradoxically you might spend more time securing their future than actually being with them.

Older dad

We value age as a source of wisdom and patience and of course it is theoretically possible to become a dad no matter how old you are. You don't even need to worry about the sweaty bit either, even if masturbation is not possible through erectile dysfunction. Prostatic massage can often produce sufficient ejaculate for assisted insemination. Finance is also usually less of a problem and your decision to have kids is less likely to be based on an irrational red haze. Smaller family size is also more likely, increasing personal contact and lessening the burden of responsibility.

Just a thought however before dispensing with the Zimmer for a few vital moments. Death, the grim reaper, is more likely to rob your children of your presence at an earlier age. You are less likely to take part in their activities and conception may be more difficult. There is also an increased risk of genetic malformation. Even so, average life expectancy is increasing and the older dad of the industrial revolution with a life expectancy of less than 40 years, is the middle-aged father of today.

Perhaps not having too much control over the matter is better in the end.

PART 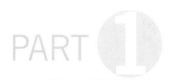 # Getting started

Is it possible to get stuck when making love?

Cramp is a dreadful invention. It always affects your calf just when you really don't want it to happen. Simply wiggling your little toe produces a pain equalled only by a meaningful relationship with Vlad the Impaler. Vaginismus is a cramp-like spasm which contracts the vagina. It is not so painful but it can be embarrassing. Some women even experience it when having a cervical smear performed. It can also occur during intercourse but the chances of endlessly doing the lambada with your trapped partner round and round the kitchen are extremely small. More important is the discomfort it can cause for both of you. Extended foreplay, which does not mean asking, 'Are you awake Sheila?' can do the trick. That and a sense of humour along with a relaxed atmosphere. But not too relaxed, you don't want to fall asleep, Sheila.

Introduction

Ovulation usually occurs somewhere between 12 and 16 days before the start of the next menstrual period. This is known as the fertile period and it is during this time that the egg can be fertilised. If your partner has regular periods, this point can be worked out with reasonable accuracy by calculating backwards from when the next period is expected. Ovulation can be detected by a change in body temperature but this indicator is usually used when trying to avoid a pregnancy as it tells you that ovulation has already occurred. A change in the degree of stickiness of the mucus on the cervix is a better indicator that ovulation is about to take place. There are self-test ovulation kits available from your pharmacist that determine when ovulation is likely to happen. These are expensive and there is little evidence that they actually increase the chance of becoming pregnant any sooner then it would happen normally. Luckily, pinpointing the exact fertile period is not necessary for most people as sperm have the ability to stay alive inside the woman for several days. Therefore sex 2-3 times a week throughout the cycle will maximise the chance of achieving a pregnancy by ensuring that sperm are ready and waiting for when the egg is released.

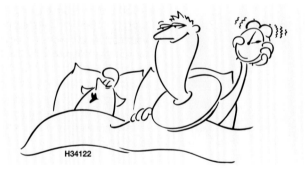

H34122

Ovulation time

Self help

There are some things you and your partner can do to help you be fit and healthy for pregnancy. Rubella infection in pregnancy can harm a developing baby, so your partner should check with her doctor to see if she needs a vaccination before you try for a pregnancy.

Women planning a baby should take 400 micrograms (0.4 mg) of folic acid every day from the time they stop using contraception until the 12th week of pregnancy, as folic acid reduces the risk of a baby having neural tube defects, such as spina bifida. (Those who have previously had a child with spina bifida or those who are taking drugs for epilepsy need to take bigger doses. Ask your doctor.) You can get folic acid from pharmacies.

A balanced diet with as much fresh food as possible will ensure enough vitamins and minerals are eaten. Soft cheeses, pâtés, soft-boiled eggs, cold prepared meats and cook-chilled foods should be avoided as there is a small risk of them being contaminated with listeria which can cause birth defects. Too much Vitamin A can be harmful to a developing baby, so pregnant women are advised not to eat liver or take Vitamin A tablets.

Your smoking Quit Plan

- Set a day and date to stop. Tell all your friends and relatives, they will support you.
- Like deep sea diving, always take a buddy. Get someone to give up with you. You will reinforce each other's will power.
- Clear the house and your pockets of any packets, papers or matches.
- One day at a time is better than leaving it open-ended.
- Map out your progress on a chart or calendar. Keep the money saved in a separate container.
- Chew on a carrot. It will help you do something with your mouth and hands.
- Ask your friends not to smoke around you. People accept this far more readily than they used to do.

Both you and your partner should try to give up smoking, as smoking is known to carry risks for the developing baby and also to newborn babies. This is just as important for men, as smokers tend to produce fewer sperm and have more damaged sperm. Quit can give you both help and advice on how to give up smoking.

Consumption of alcohol is the greatest cause of neurological damage to unborn children. When a mother drinks an excessive amount during pregnancy, Foetal Alcohol Syndrome can result. It is a pattern of mental and physical defects. It is generally agreed that alcohol in the mother's bloodstream enters the foetus by crossing the placenta. This interferes with the oxygen supply and nourishment necessary for normal cell development in the brain and other body organs.

Babies born with FAS often exhibit some if not all of the following symptoms:
- Short nose.
- Small eyes.
- Thinned upper lip.
- Small head and brain.
- Poor co-ordination.
- Hyperactivity.

It is generally believed that for the avoidance of FAS, small amounts of alcohol on a regular basis are better than irregular drinking binges. However, to keep your unborn baby safe, it is advisable **not to drink at all**. Over the page are a few simple recipes that can be as delicious as any alcoholic beverage.

Weight can affect fertility by interfering with ovulation. Women who are very underweight or overweight might want to talk to NHS Direct or their practice nurse.

Is there something wrong with masturbating when you are having regular sex?

Masturbation is subtly different from sex. First it is almost one hundred per cent safe. Most men and women in stable, happy relationships also masturbate. This is where fantasy plays its part. Many people masturbate after sex to prolong the pleasure. This is particularly noted in couples where one or other of them falls fast asleep with the final gasp with little time to ask whether the earth moved for their partner also.

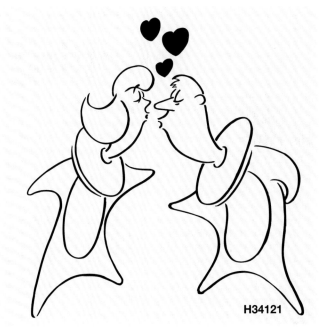

H34121

Getting started

Some sexually-transmitted infections (eg, chlamydia) can cause fertility problems, some can be passed to the baby during the pregnancy or at birth (eg, HIV) and some are thought to be linked with miscarriage or premature birth (eg, trichomonas and syphilis). Many of the infections have no symptoms so if you or your partner are worried that you may have caught a sexually-transmitted infection either recently or in the past, go to a genito-urinary medicine (GUM) clinic or sexual health clinic. The service is completely free and confidential. Most large hospitals have a GUM clinic – phone Sexual Health Direct or NHS Direct for details of your nearest clinic.

Women should avoid changing cat litter, wear gloves when gardening, and wash hands thoroughly after handling cooked meat. This prevents infection with a parasite (toxoplasmosis) which can harm a developing baby. It is also best to avoid X-rays and taking medication when you are pregnant or trying for a baby. Ask your doctor or a pharmacist if you need to do either of these.

Reducing the number of times you have sex to 'build up' a reservoir of sperm is not necessary. Sperm are produced constantly and each ejaculation contains many millions of sperm – more than enough to fertilise an egg. It is also not necessary to have sex every day, 2-3 times a week is plenty to achieve a pregnancy.

Not all couples achieve a pregnancy straight away so don't panic if it doesn't happen quickly as most couples get there within a year or so. Best just to try and be relaxed and enjoy not having to worry about contraception for a while.

Results

Testing for pregnancy is simple and accurate.

All pregnancies are followed by careful monitoring through regular visits to the doctor or midwife, ultrasound and a range of other tests where necessary, so the chances of serious problems with the birth or the baby are low.

San Francisco

Serves 1
Treat your taste buds!

3 ice cubes
1 measure orange juice
1 measure lemon juice
1 measure pineapple juice
1 measure grapefruit juice
2 dashes grenadine
1 egg white
soda water

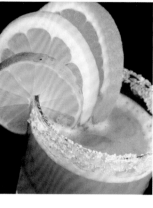

Put the ice cubes into a cocktail shaker and pour in the orange, lemon, pineapple and grapefruit juices, grenadine and egg white. Shake well then strain into a large goblet. Top up with soda water and decorate with the lemon and lime slices, a cocktail cherry on a cocktail stick and an orange spiral. Serve with a straw.

To decorate:
Lemon slice, Lime slice, Cocktail cherry, Orange spiral

Bugs Bunny

Serves 1

50 ml (2fl oz) carrot juice
50 ml (2fl oz) orange juice
4-6 ice cubes
1 dash Tabasco sauce
1 celery stick, to decorate

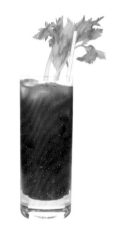

Pour the carrot and orange juices into a tumbler over ice, add a dash of Tabasco and decorate with a celery stick.

Romanov Fizz

Serves 2

8-10 ripe strawberries, hulled
125 ml (4 fl oz) orange juice
2 ice cubes
125 ml (4 fl oz) soda water

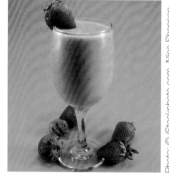

Put the strawberries and orange juice into a food processor and process until smooth. Place 1 ice cube in each of 2 sour glasses or wine glasses and add the strawberry liquid. Pour the soda water into the food processor, process briefly and use to top up the glasses. Stir briskly, and serve.

Appleade

Serves 3

2 large dessert apples
600 m (1 pint) boiling water
½ teaspoon sugar
ice cubes
apple slices, to decorate

Chop the apples and place in
a bowl. Pour the boiling water
over the apples and add the
sugar. Leave to stand for
1-2 minutes, then strain into
a jug and allow to cool. Pour over ice cubes in tall glasses and
decorate with apple slices. Serve with straws.

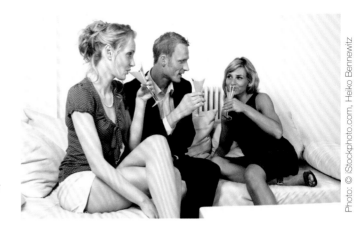

Photo: © iStockphoto.com, Heiko Bennewitz

Chocolate Shake

Serves 1

2 measures chocolate syrup
2 scoops chocolate ice cream
1 scoop vanilla ice cream
250 ml (8 fl oz) full-fat milk
whipped cream, to decorate
(optional)

Pour all of the ingredients into
a food processor. Process well
until the desired thickness is
reached. Pour into a tall glass.
Decorate with whipped cream,
if liked, and serve with straw.

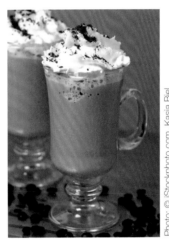

Photo: © iStockphoto.com, Kasia Biel

Keep Sober

Serves 1

½ measure grenadine
½ measure lemon syrup
3 measures tonic water
soda water
ice cubes

Put the grenadine, lemon syrup
and tonic water in a tumbler
and stir together. Top up with
soda water and add ice cubes,
if liked.

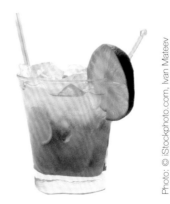

Photo: © iStockphoto.com, Ivan Mateev

Variation
For a tangier drink, replace the grenadine with lime syrup and
decorate the drink with lime slices.

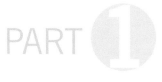
Best positions for getting pregnant

Sperm are strong swimmers, and can remain active for a few days, so any activity which places them in the vagina can result in pregnancy unless contraception is used.

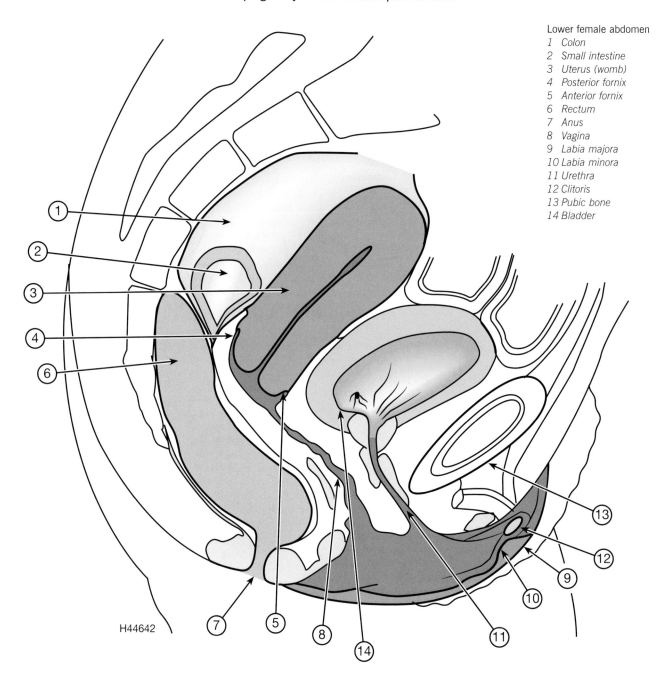

Lower female abdomen
1 Colon
2 Small intestine
3 Uterus (womb)
4 Posterior fornix
5 Anterior fornix
6 Rectum
7 Anus
8 Vagina
9 Labia majora
10 Labia minora
11 Urethra
12 Clitoris
13 Pubic bone
14 Bladder

H44642

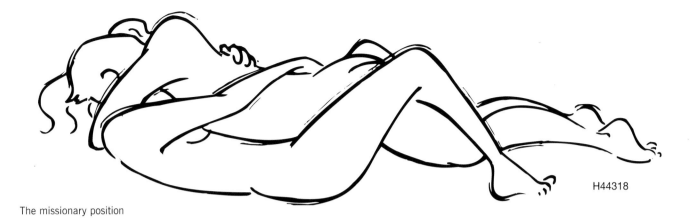

H44318

The missionary position

If the aim is to get pregnant, you can assist the sperm in their journey by using a sexual position which puts gravity to good use and positions the semen near the entry to the womb.

• The missionary position is good, especially if the woman raises her hips with a pillow and remains lying in place for 30 minutes or so after ejaculation. The same holds for any position which has the woman on her back.
• Similarly, the spoons position puts the sperm in the right place and doesn't make it run away again.
• Any variation on doggie style also puts the sperm in the right place, but it might not be so comfortable to remain in postion while gravity does its stuff.

The myth that the woman needs to have an orgasm to conceive is unproven, although it is possible that the waves which accompany an orgasm may assist in moving the sperm towards the egg.

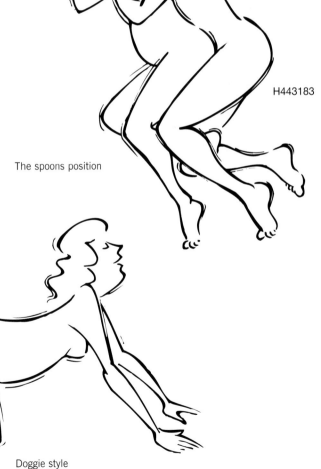

H443183

The spoons position

H39925

Doggie style

PART ① Impotence (erectile dysfunction)

Introduction

Even in these enlightened times there is still confusion over erectile dysfunction (ED/impotence) and infertility. A man can father children without being able to have an erection. Problems with erections are common. At least one in 10 British men have had some sort of erectile dysfunction at some stage in their lives. Furthermore, around one man in twenty has permanent erectile dysfunction problems. This is not helped by most men's reluctance to discuss these problems, despite the fact that virtually all of them can be overcome by relatively simple treatments.

As the penis works by hydrostatic pressure allowing blood into the spongy tissues of the penis but restricting its outflow, anything which affects the blood vessels or nerves which bring this about will influence the ability to have an erection. Unfortunately there are a large number of things which will interfere with this process, not least medicines prescribed for totally different reasons.

At one time, what was going on between a man's ears was considered the major factor for ED. We now know that around one third of all cases will be purely psychological, and will often respond well to non-clinical treatments such as sex counselling. Generally speaking, if you have erections at any other time other than during attempted intercourse then you have a psychological rather than physiological problem. Successful erections during television programmes, sexy videos or self-masturbation bode well for the future, although it is not a 100 per cent test.

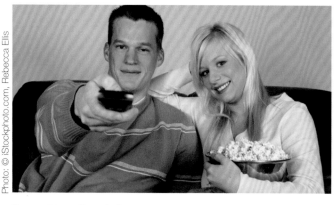

Photo: © iStockphoto.com, Rebecca Ellis

Successful erections during sexy videos bodes well for the future

When the flesh needs convincing

While there is great variation in the actual size of the penis throughout the animal kingdom, humans come top of the list in their group, the primates. (However, unlike some of the other primates we do not have prehensile tails.) For all primates the

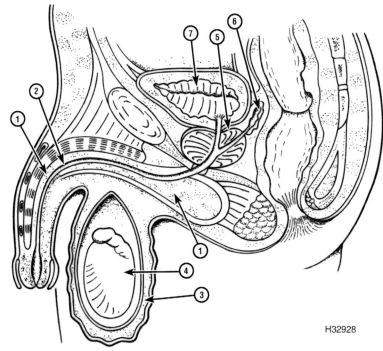

H32928

Almost half the penile structure is hidden within the pelvis
1 *Erectile tissue*
2 *Urethra*
3 *Scrotum*
4 *Testis*
5 *Prostate*
6 *Seminal vesicle*
7 *Bladder*

penis appears to have a disproportionate influence over the everyday life of the species; few other animals give sex, as distinct from reproduction, the same level of priority. Similarly, the role of the human penis is complex and extends beyond a means of transferring sperm to the female or even passing urine. Society places a certain importance on the size of a man's penis. It is said that the CIA seriously considered supplying over-sized condoms to villagers during the Vietnam/Cambodian war to enhance the 'prowess' of American troops in the eyes of the enemy.

Hydraulic system

There is no bone in the penis. Its function depends upon a hydraulic system which Citroën owners will readily understand. Just as a balloon filled with water is more rigid than one without, the erect penis uses the same principle, using blood rather than water as the stiffening medium. By allowing blood into spongy tissue within the penis, but restricting its exit, the penis can enlarge by around 2 inches during an erection.

While valuable for placing sperm well into the vagina, an erection hinders the passing of urine. Indeed there is a one-way valve at the base of the penis which prevents urine being passed at the same time as semen. Urine or sperm travel down the penis from the bladder or testes in a thin tube called the urethra.

The thin skin of the penis is covered in small bumps which may be important in stimulation of the sexual partner. Unfortunately they also cause a disproportionate amount of concern, particularly amongst young men. These are the sweat glands and hair follicles that are not normally felt on thicker skin. They are even more noticeable during an erection because the skin is stretched much thinner.

Average sizes

While men are prone to exaggerate, the average size of the human penis is around three-and-a-half to seven inches. There are operations which lengthen the penis by up to 50 per cent as almost half the penile structure is hidden within the pelvis. By cutting the ligaments which tether the penis to the pubic bones, the true length is exposed. The only serious side effect is the alteration in the angle of dangle. Instead of the erect penis standing to attention, it tends to take a more horizontal position. This is not said to adversely affect sexual pleasure. Numerous studies, however, have shown that penile length is not the main factor for sexual pleasure in the female or male partner.

A more effective and far less traumatic way of increasing penis length is to lose any excess weight.

Erectile Dysfunction (ED)

Age: the great escape

If ever there was a universal scapegoat for things that go wrong with the human body, particularly sexual activity, it has to be 'too many birthdays'. Thankfully we are realising that sex is not just for the young and the enjoyment of sex can go on indefinitely. Expressions such as 'dirty old man' are becoming less common as we all live longer and older people predominate in our society.

Age-related problems do exist, but they are by no mean the major cause. Some important facts have emerged with recent studies:

- There is a gradual decline in testosterone levels and levels of this hormone can have an effect on target organs such as the penis.

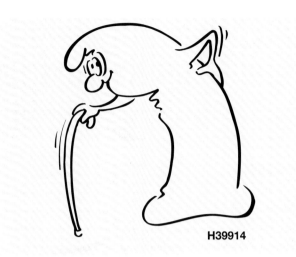

H39914

With age, erections take longer to develop and may require more tactile stimulation

- Erections take longer to develop and may require more tactile stimulation. Yes, the old Bentley may take longer to start than the new Porsche but it will give you a more comfortable ride. Might not run out of petrol so soon either.
- Self image and concerns over sexual activity tend to be problems in later life. Men are notoriously bad at confronting these problems and will often let age take the blame.
- Physical illnesses take their toll on sexual activity, not least because of the drugs which are commonly prescribed by way of treatment. We do tend to accumulate chronic conditions as we age.
- Gaps in sexual activity can be important, if only the toll they can take on sexual confidence. Bereavement, illness of the partner or divorce are good examples.
- Men are slow to admit depression to their doctors, older men even more so. Depression is a major factor for erectile dysfunction.

Common medicines and alcohol

Some medicines are known to cause problems with erections:
- Some anti-depressants are paradoxically capable of making erectile dysfunction even worse. On the other hand, some can delay premature ejaculation, which can be helpful. Talk to your doctor.
- Some anti-hypertensive drugs for high blood pressure are common culprits. ACE inhibitors, alpha and beta blockers, and calcium channel blockers can all cause problems for certain individuals. You can change your medicine to help. Talk to your doctor.
- Alcohol is a common cause. Obviously binge drinking has an immediate effect but chronic alcohol abuse can lead to permanent problems with erectile dysfunction. Small amounts of alcohol in the blood (up to 25 mg per 100 ml, or a couple of drinks in plain English) make erections easier. Any more can cause the dreaded 'droop'.
- Tobacco has an immediate short-term effect but is a much worse long-term factor. You can't have an erection when you're dead.

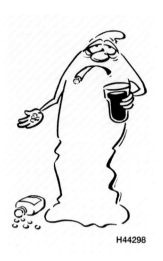

Medicines and alcohol can be a factor

Common disease culprits

Diseases which affect the nerves or blood supply can also cause problems:

- Multiple sclerosis is the commonest spinal cord disease causing erectile dysfunction. There can also be bladder problems.
- Diabetes can cause a peripheral nerve problem which affects the ability to have an erection and tends to go undiagnosed for many years.
- Vascular (blood circulation) problems account for around 25 per cent of erectile dysfunction in men. They usually have an insidious onset and are made worse by taking even small amounts of alcohol.

Diagnosis

A proper medical check-up is needed to look for any underlying cause of erectile dysfunction.

Your history will be the most important tool for diagnosis, but various tests on hormone levels are often performed.

Some diseases which travel in families, such as diabetes, hypertension or depression can also be an important clue to diagnosis. Details of drinking habits (remember brewer's droop?), smoking, diet and exercise can all be important.

Examination

A number of tests can be performed to exclude physiological causes. These include tests for:

- Diabetes.
- Anaemia.
- Liver problems.
- Thyroid deficiency (the thyroid is a gland in the neck which acts as a sort of thermostat for body metabolism. If it is set 'too low' then everything slows down, including erections).
- Testosterone, prolactin and leutenising hormone levels. The balance between all three show if you are producing the right levels of hormone to make erections possible in the first place.

Your doctor will also check:

- Blood circulation. Poor blood flow thorough arteries in your legs can also mean the same thing for your penis. Your legs use bone to stay straight, your penis can only use the pressure of blood.
- Loss of facial hair, large breasts or small testes. These all indicate a hormone problem.

Prevention

Avoiding excessive alcohol and tobacco are the obvious first lines of attack. Check with your doctor whether any drugs you are taking could be part of the problem.

Treatment

Herbal and traditional remedies are freely available but there is little evidence for their effectiveness.

Some simple treatments require a sense of humour, not least vacuum devices which have been around for over 70 years. They work by drawing blood into the penis under a gentle vacuum produced by a sheath placed over the penis and evacuated with a small pump. By restricting the blood from leaving with a tight rubber band at the base of the penis, a respectable erection can be produced. It makes sense to remove the band after 30 minutes or so to avoid problems with blood clotting. They can be used in men with vascular problems.

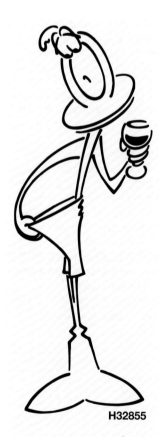

It is a golden opportunity to have a proper medical check for any underlying cause of erectile dysfunction

Psychological causes

The treatment of psychological impotence depends on education, the use of methods such as the temporary prohibition of sexual intercourse, the encouragement of touching and sensual massage (sensate focus technique) and sexual counselling.

You will need to be honest with yourself and your counsellor. They will want to know a number of important things:

- Childhood experiences and your attitude to sexuality. This may well include the attitudes of your partner.
- Your sexual experience during adolescence.
- Your own body image and how you feel about your genitals.
- How content you are with your sexual relationships.
- 'Bad trips'. Have you had some painful experiences which are flavouring your appreciation of sex.
- Your feelings about sexual arousal. What is 'normal' or 'acceptable' practice.
- How you rate yourself as a sexual being.

After looking into these areas they will want to know if these problems came on suddenly, and what preceded them. Psychological problems tend to come on quite abruptly whereas physiological causes tend to be more insidious. Your medical history will be examined. Some drugs (medicinal and recreational) can cause erectile problems. Even homeopathic treatments can be a factor.

Oral treatments

The great leap forward came with oral preparations which are increasing in number, mode of action, duration of action and safety. They allow as near as possible 'normal' sex but still require stimulation and arousal as they are not aphrodisiacs.

Although around 80% of men will be able to get an erection adequate for intercourse with drug support, probably less than half will continue with therapy in the longer term. The likely reason for this is that both doctors and their male patients tend to focus on erection and genital function rather than on sexual satisfaction, and this is a very personal factor. A rigid erection alone will not necessarily help you talk comfortably and openly about your sexual fantasies and ideas, particularly if you have not had sex for a long time.

Couples using drug therapies need ongoing support and encouragement until they are satisfied with the outcome of treatment. It is important that you understand how to use the drugs properly as nearly one third of men who failed to get adequate erections with a drug could do so when re-instructed on its proper use.

Another important issue is that, whether using drug therapy or not, older men take longer to get an erection and often require direct genital stimulation to do so. Some men believe that their inability to get an erection through fantasy or visual stimulation alone is abnormal, whereas it should really be expected with ageing. Variety really can be quite literally the spice of life here and more variety in sexual behaviour can be helpful. Cuddling, play and talking are all part of the sex act which will have gone as well so needs to be put back into practice.

Injections

Hormone injections straight into the penis may be a better option. The needle is so fine it is virtually painless but you need to inject into different places to stop any scarring.

Injections of drugs straight into the spongy tissue of the penis

can mimic the way the nerves work by restricting the blood flow out of the penis, thus producing an erection in men with these problems. It is surprisingly free of pain, although most men cross their legs just thinking about it.

These treatments can be effective in men who have not responded to oral therapies, but they may not always be acceptable to men or their partners. Unlike oral therapies, they provoke erection directly without the need for external stimulation.

Penile implants

If there is no response to injections, a penile prosthesis may be the answer. Before you go down this road both you and your partner need to understand what is involved. There is a certain sacrifice of dignity which both of you will need to come to terms with. Having said that, many couples find the release of sexual frustration far outweighs the temporary embarrassment.

There are three versions of implantable devices:

- Semi-rigid rods, made of silicone, sometimes covered with stainless steel braiding, are inserted into the spongy tissue of the penis.
- Two self-contained cylinder pumps are inserted into the penis and filled by squeezing a reservoir in the base of the penis.
- Inflatable penis prostheses consist of a pair of inflatable silicone cylinders implanted in the penis which can be filled by squeezing a pump implanted in the scrotum.

They all work. But as the old saying goes, 'it's not the size, it's what you do with it that counts'. Foreplay, sexual experimentation, avoidance of routine and being honest with each other is just as important as having a functional erection. Oh yes, and a healthy dollop of a sense of humour too. Sex after all is not only enjoyable, it can be good fun as well.

Does having sex on an aeroplane make your testicles blow up?

Fortunately not. Otherwise it would give terrorists a whole new dimension to plane hijacks. Members of the Mile High Club, an exclusive group of underweight individuals who loiter around airborne toilets, are particularly happy. 'You are aware of something which doesn't happen on the ground' one leading member who wishes to remain anonymous told me, 'perhaps it is the reduced cabin pressure'. More likely the cabin crew adjusting the video camera for the next office party. If you take a plastic mineral water bottle on board it will fizz far more on opening as the cabin pressure is maintained as the equivalent of that at a few thousand feet. This has no effect on the internal organs, or the external ones for that matter. Newton's law states, however, that to every action there is an equal and opposite reaction so you might like to tell your Mile High Partner to adopt the brace position.

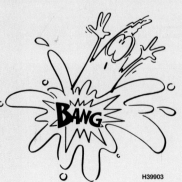

H39903

PART **1**

Technical specs for pregnancy

Technically, and by definition, pregnancy starts at the moment a sperm penetrates an egg. For practical reasons the start of pregnancy is taken from the first day of the last menstrual period, rather than from the date of fertilisation. Labour and the delivery of the baby can be expected 280 days (40 weeks) from the start of the last period. The length of pregnancy may, however, vary between about 37 and 42 weeks. This variation is the constant cause for more fear, angst and superstition than just about anything else to do with pregnancy.

Sperms can carry either an X chromosome or a Y chromosome. If an X fertilises, the result will be a girl; if Y the result will be a boy. Sperms and eggs each contain 23 chromosomes. This is half the full number. So when a sperm and an egg fuse, the full complement of chromosomes is made up, and fertilisation is said to have occurred, giving the normal 46 chromosomes. Some genetic defects are linked to extra or missing chromosomes.

In a normal body cell, there are 46 chromosomes containing

Sperms and eggs can carry an X or Y chromosome

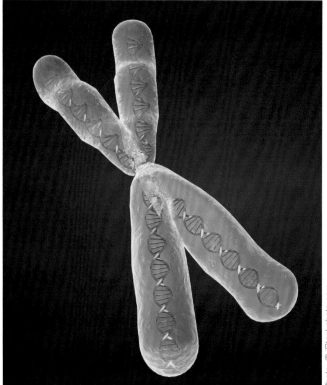

Photo: © iStockphoto.com

all the genetic information and arranged in 23 pairs. One set of 23 comes from the father, the other set from the mother. A fertilised ovum (egg) with its 23 pairs of chromosomes, starts to divide, rapidly and repeatedly. Every time a cell divides and reproduces, the 46 chromosomes are copied precisely.

Humans generally produce one baby at a time but sometimes after the first division the cells will separate to produce two individuals with exactly the same chromosomes. These are identical twins. Very rarely, this may happen again to one of the eggs, producing identical triplets.

Fertilisation usually occurs in the fallopian tube which connects the womb to the ovary and the resulting embryo passes into the womb and begins to implant into the womb inner lining (see *Ectopic pregnancy* on page 39). At once the embryo sends out tiny finger-like processes called chorionic villi which help to anchor it into the womb lining and which later become the placenta.

Very soon, usually within one week, these villi are producing a hormone called human chorionic gonadotrophin. This prevents the body from going through menstruation which would end the pregnancy.

At ten weeks, the baby is about the size of your little toe and has all the recognisable external characteristics of a human male or female. At this stage the face is formed but the eyelids are fused together. The brain is in a very primitive state.

After three months, the baby is as long as your little finger.

In the sixth month, the baby is longer than your middle finger and weighs up to 800 g. Survival outside of the womb is very unlikely. The chances of survival increase rapidly with increasing maturity and most babies over 1000 g (1 kg) now do well in an intensive care ward.

The womb (uterus) steadily grows with the baby and eventually rises inside the abdomen. The baby is surrounded by a fluid-filled double membrane, the inner layer of which is called the amnion. The membrane normally ruptures and releases the amniotic fluid ('breaking of the waters') before the baby is born.

Around one litre of amniotic fluid fills the womb in which the baby floats freely. This fluid is protective and is constantly swallowed and then excreted as urine by the baby, so it contains material from which much information about the health of the baby can be obtained. Samples can be obtained through a needle in the procedure called amniocentesis (see page 43).

The placenta is a thick, disc-shaped object about the size of your hand. The mother's blood enters the placenta from the womb side and the umbilical cord comes off from the free surface. In the placenta, the maternal blood comes into close contact with, but does not mix with, the foetal blood, which is being pumped through the placenta by the foetal heart.

A large number of nutrients and gases such as oxygen, carbon dioxide, sugars, amino acids, fats, vitamins, minerals, as well as many drugs, pass freely across the placental barrier. It is in this way that the baby is provided with all necessary supplies for maintenance as well as for body growth, and is able to get rid of waste substances.

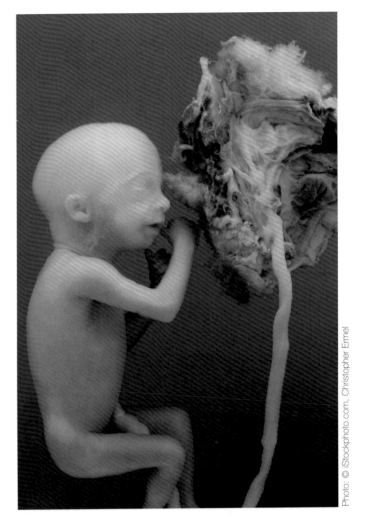

PART **1**

Artificial insemination and IVF

The term artificial insemination sounds daunting and cold. Some fertility clinics call it intra-uterine insemination for this very reason. Whatever it is called, it is actually a simple way of becoming pregnant if it is very difficult or impossible to manage it through sexual intercourse. If that does not work, more sophisticated treatments are available.

Note that impotence (erectile dysfunction/ED) and infertility are not the same thing. A man can be unable to have an erection yet be perfectly capable of having children by treating the erectile dysfunction (see *Impotence* on page 24) or by using assisted methods of conception. Sub-fertility, where there are too few sperm in the semen, or they are not able to swim correctly, does not necessarily mean that you cannot have children.

In cases of erectile dysfunction, seminal fluid can often be obtained by masturbation or by massaging the prostate under an anaesthetic. This is called AIP (artificial insemination by partner). With reduced fertility (sub-fertility) pregnancy can sometimes be achieved by placing the semen directly into the cervix. With severely reduced fertility, semen can be provided by another man. This is called AID (artificial insemination by donor). Most donors remain anonymous although the law is being pressed on this issue should your child wish to know their 'natural' father. You need to discuss this fully with your partner and medical staff.

Many couples (and single women) decide to go down the do it yourself insemination route, it isn't difficult. There are many websites with advice and instructions, just use an Internet search engine. Basically it involves collecting semen produced by masturbation and using a syringe (without a needle) to put it in the vagina.

Of course any form of artificial insemination carries connotations and must always be second best, but it is relatively easy, quick and results in the vast majority of cases in a perfectly normal baby.

Is there a problem?

Out of every ten couples trying for children eight achieve pregnancy within a year, one couple will conceive within two years and the remaining couple will need medical help. Many doctors will not consider referring a couple for infertility investigations until they have been trying for around two years (one year if the couple are over 35 years old).

How long you should spend trying for pregnancy before seeking help depends to some extent on the medical histories and age of you and your partner. Consult your GP or attend a family planning clinic for women if your partner:

● Has irregular periods, or the menstrual cycle is shorter than 21 or longer than 35 days.
● Finds intercourse painful.
● Has a history of pelvic inflammatory disease.
● Has had any abdominal surgery.
● Has a history of chlamydia or another sexually transmitted infection.
● Is underweight or overweight.
● Is aged over 35.

Consult your GP or attend a family planning clinic for men if you:
● Have had an operation on the testes, or had treatment for testicular cancer or an undescended testicle.
● Have a history of chlamydia or another sexually transmitted infection.
● Have a history of mumps after puberty.
● Are very overweight.
Be prepared to discuss questions such as:
● Your general medical health.
● Your partner's menstrual cycle.
● Previous methods of contraception.
● Any previous pregnancies/miscarriages/abortions.
● Any infections, including sexually transmitted infections.
● How often you have intercourse.

Causes of infertility and possible treatments

A woman who has difficulty in ovulating may need a course of drugs.

A woman not producing eggs may need another woman to donate eggs (this is not routinely offered).

A woman with blocked fallopian tubes may need surgery or assisted conception.

A man with a low count and/or poor quality of sperm may need assisted conception to aid fertilisation using his own sperm. Alternatively, sperm from a donor may be needed.

There may be other, less common, causes and a couple may have a combination of problems, so investigations need to be completed even if one problem is found at an early stage. Most problems can be helped, with varying degrees of success. Sometimes, even after full investigations, the reason for infertility cannot be found but assisted conception treatment may still be successful.

Visiting your GP gives you and your partner the opportunity to ask about the possible investigations and treatments, waiting lists and any costs. You can then decide if you want to go ahead with

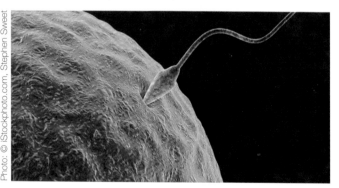
Photo: © iStockphoto.com, Stephen Sweet

tests and/or treatment. You will want to know what treatments are offered locally on the NHS and, if you wish to consider paying for private treatment, what private treatments are available locally. You should also find out whether the NHS will meet the costs of any prescribed drugs or if you will have to pay for them.

While GPs can do some preliminary investigations, you may need to be referred to a specialist fertility clinic. If so, you will need a referral letter from your GP. The provision of specialist services within the NHS is limited in some areas and waiting lists vary for certain types of treatment, so try to find out how long you are likely have to wait for an appointment.

Eligibility for NHS treatment

The type of treatment you can receive on the NHS depends on a number of factors, including what infertility services local health services decide they will purchase.

Some patients will be investigated and treated at their local hospital, others may be referred on to a specialist unit. There is often a limit on the amount of treatment you can receive.

While most tests and investigations are carried out on the NHS, around 80 per cent of in-vitro fertilisation (IVF) treatment is carried out privately. You need to find out what the funding and selection criteria are to see if you will be eligible for NHS treatment. You could also contact the Human Fertilisation and Embryology Authority (HFEA) for a copy of its Patients' Guide to clinics. The reputations and success rates of different fertility clinics vary widely. If venturing outside the NHS, be wary of fraudulent practitioners – check on the HFEA website.

Fertility tests

A specialist clinic will be able to carry out many different kinds of tests to see what the problem is and to find out which treatments will be best for you.

Clinics offer different types of treatment, and no single clinic is going to be best for everyone. Practical factors such as the opening times, the costs, the length of the clinic's waiting list and the travelling involved are also important.

The kind of tests that are done vary from clinic to clinic. Once you have a diagnosis, fairly simple treatment or surgery may be all that is needed. Not all of the following tests may be necessary, but they include:

- **Semen analysis** to look at the number, shape and size of sperm and how well they move. More than one test should be carried out.
- **Blood or urine tests** to check hormone levels.
- **X-rays/scans** to find blockages or check blood supply to the testes.
- **Blood, urine and cervical mucus checks** to verify hormone levels or detect ovulation.
- **Ultrasound scans** to check if a follicle, which should contain an egg, is being produced. Treatment for ovulation problems usually involves drugs by tablets, injections or nasal inhalations – and has a high success rate if the correct diagnosis has been established.
- **Sperm mucus crossover** – this checks if the woman's cervical mucus allows her partner's sperm through.
- **Endometrial biopsy** – a tiny sample of womb lining (endometrium) is removed to check that it is free from infection and that ovulation has occurred.
- **Hysterosalpingogram** where dye is passed through the fallopian tubes to check that they are open and clear of obstruction.
- **Laparoscopy** (usually under general anaesthetic) uses a thin

telescope-like instrument to view the female reproductive organs through a small cut below the navel. It checks for scar tissue, endometriosis, fibroids or any abnormality in the shape or position of the womb, ovaries or fallopian tubes. At the same time a dye may be passed through the fallopian tubes to see if they are open and clear.

Assisted conception

Assisted conception techniques have been used successfully for many years and a range of techniques is available. It is now possible for some men with very low sperm counts or even with no sperm in their semen to have their own genetic children. A specialist clinic will be able to advise you on which treatment will be best for you.

The most well-known treatment is in-vitro fertilisation (IVF) in which eggs are removed from the woman, fertilised in the laboratory and the embryo is then placed into her womb. Others include:

- **Donor Insemination (DI)** uses sperm from anonymous donor, where there are severe problems with the man's sperm.
- **Gamete Intra-Fallopian Transfer (GIFT)** uses a couple's own eggs and sperm, or those of donors, which are mixed together and placed in the woman's fallopian tubes where they fertilise.
- **Intra-Cytoplasmic Sperm Injection (ICSI)** uses a single sperm injected into the woman's egg which is then transferred to the womb after fertilisation.

These are not miracle solutions. The age of your partner is very important. A woman aged under 35 has a much better chance of a successful pregnancy than one over 40.

Donor insemination (DI) of sperm and donor eggs

If a man produces no or few normal sperm, carries an inherited disease, or has had a vasectomy, then insemination using sperm from an anonymous donor may be considered. Egg donation may be an option if a woman is not producing eggs or has a genetic problem. The decision to use donor sperm or eggs can be a difficult one. You can get help in making this decision from a counsellor or support group.

Clinics which offer this service have to send information about donors, recipients and the outcome of treatment to the HFEA. Donors have to meet extensive screening criteria, including HIV testing. A man may not usually donate sperm after ten live births have resulted from his semen donations. Donors do not have to be anonymous and most clinics will accept a donor who a couple have found for themselves.

Counselling and support

Couples report that the many hospital visits needed and the time spent waiting between treatments to learn if each stage has worked is stressful. All units providing IVF and other licensed conception techniques have a legal responsibility to offer counselling. Counselling can allow you to talk through what the treatment entails and how you feel about it, and can give support during the process and if the treatment fails.

If you don't want to see a counsellor at the clinic you are attending, the British Infertility Counsellors Association can put you in touch with your nearest infertility counsellor. Some people find being in contact with others in a similar situation or with a support group helps them through infertility.

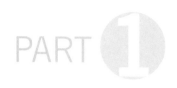

PART ①

Confirmation of pregnancy

Testing for pregnancy used to involve rabbits. Things have progressed and now the tests depend on the presence of human chorionic gonadotrophin (see *Technical specs for pregnancy* on page 28). This hormone is produced by the developing embryo and is first present in the blood, but soon afterwards appears in the urine. A simple dipstick test into fresh urine can detect pregnancy with about a 98 per cent certainty from the time of the first missed period. There are even more sensitive immunological tests which can confirm pregnancy within a week of conception. These are normally done in a hospital laboratory and are usually used when a woman has had fertility treatment. If these tests are positive the accuracy is nearly 100 per cent certain; if the test is negative, about 80 per cent certain.

Pregnancy testing kits are available over-the-counter from pharmacies. (Some pharmacies will do the test for you, which can be cheaper than buying a whole testing kit.) The important thing about home testing kits is that the instructions are followed carefully otherwise you can get a wrong result. Free pregnancy testing is also available at most GPs, family planning clinics and NHS Walk-in centres.

A missed period is a common sign of pregnancy (however it is not the only reason women miss periods). Other signs and symptoms of pregnancy are tiredness, hunger, nausea and vomiting, frequently passing urine, changes in the breasts and low abdominal pain like a period pain. Many women can tell they are pregnant even before they have had a test performed or have missed a period.

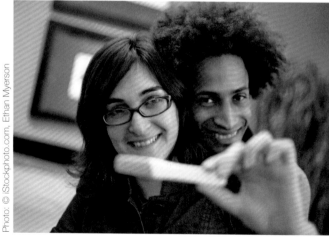

Photo: © iStockphoto.com, Ethan Myerson

PART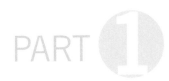

Mum's having a baby

Teens don't want to think about parents having sex – and now the reality is being forced on them! What will their friends say? How will it change their lives? A new sibling is quite a different proposition for a teenager than it is for a toddler or pre-teen. Gauging how an older – possibly wiser – teenager will react to the news calls for forethought. It really depends on the individual.

The news may come as a shock at first but don't anticipate a negative reaction. Some girls are already becoming maternal at this age, and even boys are developing a soft streak for little kids – teens often end up secretly excited, and a tiny baby isn't a threat to their status as a 'senior' member of the family.

Tell your teenagers before the world knows

Bear in mind that they are quick on the uptake. It's especially important if you're suffering from morning sickness or feeling very tired – one worried teenager's unexpected reaction to the announcement of a forthcoming sibling was 'Thank God for that, I thought you were dying!' It's better that the news comes from you rather than via someone else, so tell them before they hear it from others.

A forthcoming baby in the household is usually the last thing a teenager expects to deal with, so understand that they may be taken aback. An obvious sign of parental fertility (and everything that goes with it) is not what most teens are ready for. Your child will probably be unsure about how to feel or act. Part of them may feel excited at the news, while another part is anxious and concerned.

A new baby can be reassuring, as it makes it clear that a young person's parents are very clearly still 'together'. If it's a step-sibling it can be more upsetting. Does it mean you'll love them less? Will you devote all your time to your new family? As a parent, especially if it's your first baby with your new partner, you will be readjusting to your new relationships too. Amidst the many distractions, find time to listen to your teenagers.

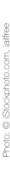

Photo: © iStockphoto.com, jallfree

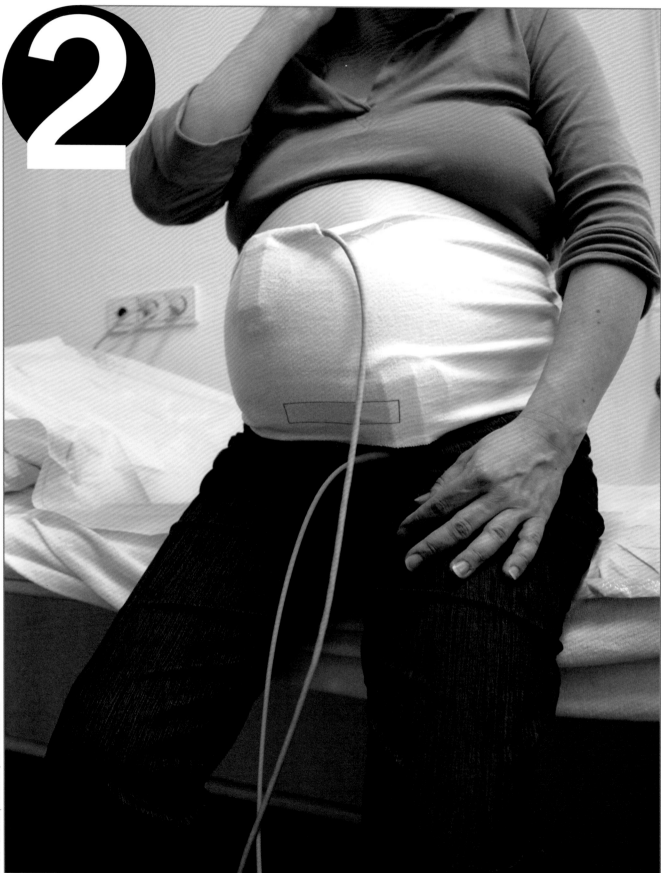

2

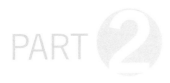

PART **2**

BABY MANUAL

Stages, monitoring and complications of pregnancy

PART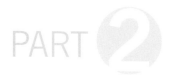

Pregnancy

Introduction

Morning sickness is not always a feature of pregnancy. Although many women suffer some nausea and vomiting in early pregnancy, this doesn't necessarily occur in the mornings. It also varies greatly in severity and may be seriously disabling, but it usually settles by about twelve weeks. Very severe vomiting may necessitate admission to hospital to replace fluids and halt the vomiting with safe medicines.

There are other aspects of pregnancy well recognised by most women, such as:

- Increased need to pass water. (Always ask your partner before she gets in the car.)
- Tiredness, sometimes severe. (Don't take it personally when she dozes off during a conversation.)

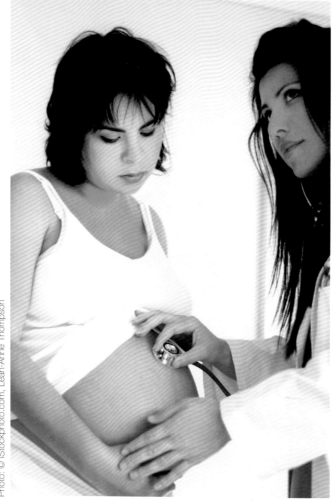

Photo: © iStockphoto.com, Lean-Anne Thompson

- Tender and/or sore breasts. (Don't touch!)
- Browning of the pink zones round the nipples (areolae).
- Linea nigra - a brown line down the belly. This will fade after pregnancy.
- 'Quickening', a perception by the mother of foetal movements generally at about the eighteenth week in a first pregnancy, and about two weeks earlier in later pregnancies.

Stages of pregnancy (trimesters)

Pregnancy is divided up into three stages of three months each called trimesters. These are completely arbitrary and for the benefit of doctors and midwives rather than potential parents. Most important basic development takes place during the first trimester so infections, radiation or harmful drugs tend to have the greatest potential for harm.

By the end of the first trimester the fingers, toes, external genitalia, facial features and ears are visible. During the second trimester, the foetal heart can be heard using a stethoscope, and midwives can generally feel the baby through the abdominal wall. Obviously all this development produces pressure on organs found in the abdomen, particularly the gut and bladder, so heart burn and frequent trips to the toilet are a feature of later stages of pregnancy. Upward pressure on the diaphragm prevents it from moving downwards fully during respiration and this limits full expansion of the lungs. For this reason a heavily pregnant woman will often suffer breathlessness.

Fleeting contractions called Braxton-Hicks contractions generally start around this time although in first time pregnancies they may be 'missed' until later on. They are perfectly normal and do not imply that labour is starting. During the second trimester the developed foetal organs begin to function, During

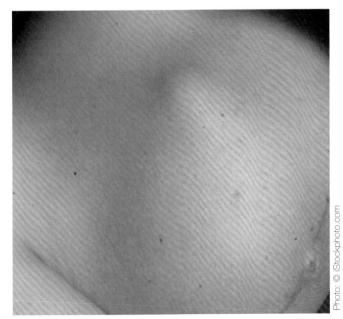

By the 7th month the baby will definitely make its presence felt! Note the linea nigra running down the belly

The baby generally lies head down, facing back (the occipito anterior position)

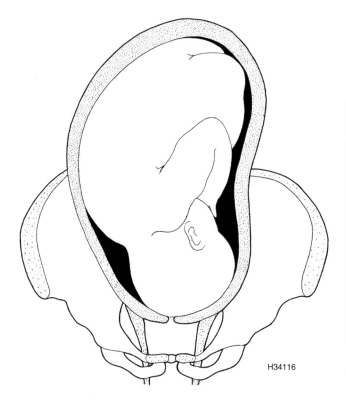

H34116

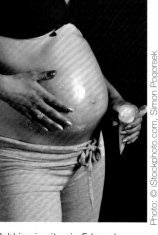

Rubbing in vitamin E based creams may help reduce stretch marks

It's a good idea for fathers to read to their babies while they are still in the womb. This will give the baby reassurance and comfort after it is born as it will recognise both its father's and mother's voice.

this second trimester the bones become more solid and are easily seen on ultrasound scanning.

During the last month of the pregnancy many women in their first pregnancy experience a sense of relief from the symptoms caused by abdominal fullness. This occurs because the baby is normally lying head-down and it may move downwards as its head sinks naturally into the pelvis. This sense of relief from abdominal pressure is called lightening. Now the mother's diaphragm is able to descend more fully and the lungs to expand so that breathing is easier. The cost of this, however, is that the pressure on the bladder and rectum may be worse. Lightening may not occur with second or subsequent pregnancies. In these, it is quite common for the baby's head to fail to 'engage' until labour has actually started.

Complications

Pregnancy is not a disease and pregnant women are not automatically ill. Similarly, the vast majority of pregnancies are event-free and have little or no problems (see the following Sections).

Even so, some things change after a pregnancy, occasionally for a long time or forever. Stretch marks, medically known as striae, are broad lines on the skin of the abdomen, thighs and breasts that affect about 70% of all pregnant women. At first red and slightly raised, they later become purplish and flattened.

Although stretch marks are thought to be caused by the stretching of the skin and the resulting damage to the elastic protein collagen in the skin, it is generally only seen where this stretching takes place because of pregnancy and may reflect hormonal changes as well. Some people feel creams containing vitamin E along with vitamin supplements in the diet can help, but the evidence is thin on the ground.

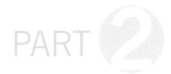

PART

Ectopic pregnancy

Introduction

A dangerous complication of pregnancy occurs when the fertilised egg (ovum) becomes implanted in an abnormal site inside the body instead of in the womb lining. The great majority of these ectopic pregnancies, over 95 per cent, occur in a fallopian tube connecting the ovaries to the womb.

Unfortunately there has been a large increase in ectopic pregnancies in the last 30 years, from about 4 per 1000 pregnancies in 1970 to about 20 per 1000. Chlamydia, a sexually-transmitted infection, is a major factor as there has been a corresponding increase in infection with this bacterium which causes pelvic inflammatory disease (PID), leading to inflammation and narrowing of the fallopian tubes.

Early diagnosis of ectopic pregnancy is vital as it can cause severe internal bleeding and further damage to the fallopian tubes, not to mention endangering the life of the woman.

Symptoms

The symptoms of ectopic pregnancy can mimic appendicitis, but usually start with cramping period-like pains and slight vaginal bleeding occurring soon after the first missed period.

Causes

Around half of all women operated on for ectopic pregnancy have evidence of pelvic inflammatory disease, the basic cause of which is often chlamydial infection.

Diagnosis

Suspicion is raised by the symptoms and a positive pregnancy test. The diagnosis is confirmed by ultrasound scanning, usually through the vagina, or by direct examination through a viewing tube passed through a small opening in the wall of the abdomen (laparoscopy).

Prevention

It is impossible to prevent an ectopic pregnancy with absolute certainty. Condoms give almost 100% protection from chlamydia infection, the single greatest cause.

Complications

Thanks to swift medical care relatively few women will die from an ectopic pregnancy, but it leaves scars on the fallopian tube which further reduce the chance of a successful pregnancy. Many women are deeply worried by the thought of future pregnancy.

Treatment

Urgent hospital management is needed. Treatment is by operation to remove the growing embryo. This is mainly done by laparoscopic surgery.

Action

Ectopic pregnancy needs immediate medical attention in an A&E/ER department. Dial 999/112.

PART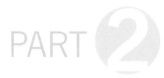

Eclampsia

Introduction
Once the scourge of pregnancy, eclampsia is now not only rare but also treatable when caught early (but potentially life-threatening if not detected). It is a disorder originating in the placenta that, once under way, causes widespread upset of the functioning of the circulatory system of both mother and baby.

Diagnosis
The most important signs of eclampsia are a significant rise in blood pressure, and the presence of the protein albumin in the urine, which will be detected by the GP or midwife. Other signs include swelling of the feet or hands and excessive weight gain.

Treatment
Rest in bed is an important measure. Drugs to reduce blood pressure are avoided, if possible, as they may interfere with the supply to the foetus through the placenta. Established eclampsia needs urgent treatment to sedate the mother, get the blood pressure down and deliver the baby as soon as possible.

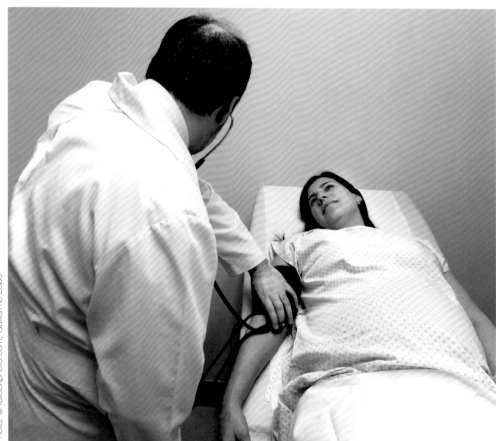

Photo: © iStockphoto.com, Guillermo Lobo

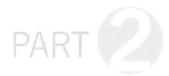

PART **Infectious diseases**

Chicken pox

If a pregnant woman comes into contact with someone who has chicken pox, she is probably immune if she has had it herself, but it is worth having a blood test to check.

● Before 20 weeks into the pregnancy. If the mother has no immunity she should have the man-made antibodies Varicella-Zoster Ig (VZ-Ig) no less than 10 days after exposure.

● Between 20 weeks and just before term. There is no risk to the baby, although the mother can get chicken pox pneumonia.

● Between one week before delivery and a month after. If the mother develops a rash during this time it is possible she hasn't passed the antibodies to the baby, who is at risk from infection.

German measles (rubella)

Although German measles (rubella) is a relatively mild and harmless viral infection in children or adults, it can have devastating effects on the early pregnancy. The more serious effects on the developing baby include:

● Heart defects.
● Cataracts.
● Deafness.
● Neurological defects.
● Mental retardation.
● Bone and joint defects.

Although the severity of effect varies greatly, with many children suffering no apparent harm, around a quarter of babies infected while in the womb will show some problems by the age of two years. Women who are not immune should be particularly careful to avoid contact with any possible case and should be immunised as soon as the pregnancy is over.

Such is the danger of malformation, any non-immune pregnant women developing a rash and swollen glands in the back of the neck early in pregnancy should get themselves checked to discover whether the condition is rubella. Termination is an option and needs discussion with professionals who can give you the facts objectively. Obviously all girls and boys should be immunised to prevent this happening in the first place.

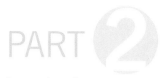

PART 2 **Miscarriage**

Introduction

Losing the baby before the 28th week of pregnancy is called a spontaneous miscarriage and occurs most commonly during the first three months of pregnancy.

It is unfortunately more common than most people think. There is still a reluctance to discuss these things openly. At least one pregnancy in ten ends in miscarriage, most of these occurring at an early stage. In many of these cases, the woman concerned is never aware that she is pregnant and experiences a late, and perhaps unusually severe, period.

Signs of miscarriage

Recognising that something has gone wrong is not always easy and people can make mistakes in both directions. Any pain in the abdomen, particularly if it is associated with blood loss from the vagina, needs to be investigated. Simply a lack of movement or just a 'feeling' that something is wrong can be a sign. Many relatively minor conditions can mimic these symptoms. Urinary tract infections (cystitis) can often cause abdominal pain and even some blood in the urine. Even the pain of constipation has been mistaken for the onset of a miscarriage. More obvious and severe lower abdominal pain suggests a possible pregnancy outside the womb (ectopic pregnancy).

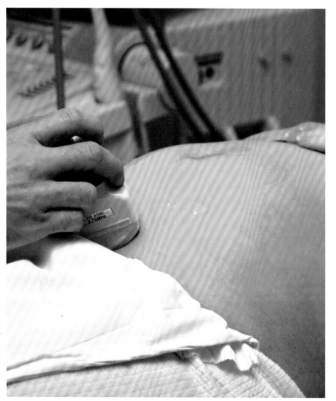

Photo: © iStockphoto.com

Causes

In the vast majority of cases there will be no obvious cause but there are some well-recognised factors such as:
- An ectopic (see *Ectopic pregnancy* on page 39) or unsuitable site in the womb for the baby to develop normally.
- An abnormality inside the womb.
- Instability of the neck of the womb which may open too soon (incompetent cervix). This affects about one pregnancy in a hundred and causes repeated, painless, spontaneous miscarriages around the fourth or fifth month of pregnancy.
- Any hormone imbalance which affects the pregnancy.
- A GU (genito urinary) infection.

Prevention

Miscarriage from incompetent cervix can often be avoided by inserting a temporary encircling stitch (a Shirodkar suture). Some of the other causes can also be treated or avoided; ask your GP for advice.

Treatment

If the miscarriage is missed or incomplete, a minor operation, under general anaesthesia, may be needed. Suction is used to clear the womb, and the lining is carefully scraped with a sharp-edged spoon called a curette. A drug is then given to cause the womb to contract, and antibiotics may also be necessary. The woman is usually able to go home the next day.

Miscarriage later in pregnancy is less common and is often associated with abnormalities of the womb or with inability of the cervix to remain closed (cervical incompetence). Full gynaecological investigation will reveal the cause of this in about 40 per cent of cases. Support from yourself along with good medical advice is needed. Generally the woman will be scanned by ultrasound (a painless, harmless, examination using sound waves which pass though skin).

Relatives may mistakenly try to be positive with comments like 'there must have been something wrong with the baby' or 'you can always try again' What is forgotten is that you and your partner are already grieving. While it is true that major abnormalities can lead to loss of the baby, we still know precious little about the process of spontaneous abortion and why apparently perfectly normal pregnancies come to an early end. Suggesting to your partner that she may have produced an abnormal baby will not help for the next pregnancy. You should recognise her need to grieve and to supply emotional support accordingly. Unfortunately, people may forget your own suffering. You too will be grieving but people may not realise. This is particularly true when there have been a number of miscarriages or if you have been trying for a long time. There are counsellors available for men as well as women and the maternity unit will put you in touch with them.

Repeated miscarriages (more than three without a successful pregnancy) should be investigated.

PART 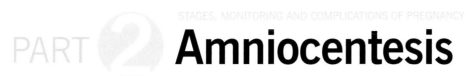 # Amniocentesis

Introduction

Along with ultrasound examination and CVS, amniocentesis is an important way of finding out how a baby is developing while inside the womb, and especially checking for any genetic abnormality. Routine amniocentesis is generally only recommended for women over 35 years old because at that age the risk of the procedure causing a miscarriage is about the same as the risk of the baby having Down's syndrome. More children with Down's syndrome are now born to younger women than previously. In other cases, amniocentesis is done if there is any special reason to suspect trouble. The risk of causing miscarriage by amniocentesis is about 0.5 per cent.

Why it is necessary

Amniocentesis provides direct information about the likelihood or certainty of the baby developing one of a number of conditions. Disorders that can be detected or strongly suspected following amniocentesis include:

- Rhesus factor disease ('blue babies').
- Serious disorders in brain development (anencephaly).
- Respiratory distress syndrome where the child has serious difficulties breathing at birth.

- Spina bifida.
- Down's syndrome.
- Cystic fibrosis.
- Haemophilia (a deficiency in blood clotting factors).
- Duchenne muscular dystrophy (a progressive muscular weakness).
- Thalassaemia (a blood disorder).
- Sickle-cell anaemia (a blood disorder which can cause clots to form in joints).
- Antitrypsin deficiency (a digestive disorder).
- Phenylketonuria (a block in the formation of an important enzyme which can cause brain damage early in life).

The amniotic fluid in which the baby floats always contains cells which drift off from the baby. These can be cultured so that chromosomes can be checked after two or three weeks. In this way a range of genetic diseases can be diagnosed before birth.

Why it should be done

Amniocentesis is a method of detecting serious or potentially serious disorders in the future child. It gives parents the option of deciding whether or not they want to have a child that will have one of these disorders, or whether they would prefer the pregnancy to be terminated at that early stage. Early treatment of some disorders while the baby remains in the womb is becoming increasingly possible.

When it should be done

Amniocentesis is usually done at or after 15 weeks into the pregnancy, most commonly between the 16th and 20th weeks. It can be done earlier than 15 weeks, but this is avoided if possible because of the greater risk of causing miscarriage or causing damage to the baby.

How it is performed

After anaesthetising a small area of the abdominal wall with a local injection, ultrasound scanning is used to guide a needle safely through the wall of the womb into the amniotic fluid in which the baby is floating. A sample of fluid can now be sucked out with a syringe. This fluid contains cells which drift off from the skin of the baby and various substances secreted by the foetus which can used for diagnosis. Every cell contains a complete set of the DNA of the baby, thus containing vital information about its development.

What happens afterwards

Your partner will be told to take things easy for a few days and to watch for any signs of possible miscarriage.

There follows a nerve-wracking wait of up to 2 weeks before the results of the test are obtained. This can be a particularly stressful time for your partner.

If the results of the test do show some abnormality, the implications will be explained to you by a specialist.

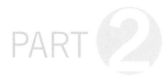

PART

Ultrasound

Introduction

Incredible advances have taken place over the past 40 years when it comes to monitoring the development of the unborn baby. Ultrasound scanning has become increasingly important as a way of scanning without using any radiation such as X-rays.

How it is done

A beam of 'sound' at a frequency of about three to ten million cycles per second is sent into the abdomen above the uterus using a machine which looks like a hand-held scanner used for computers. Tissues of different density produce echoes which return to the machine. In this way a picture of the inside of the body can be created. To make sure there is good contact

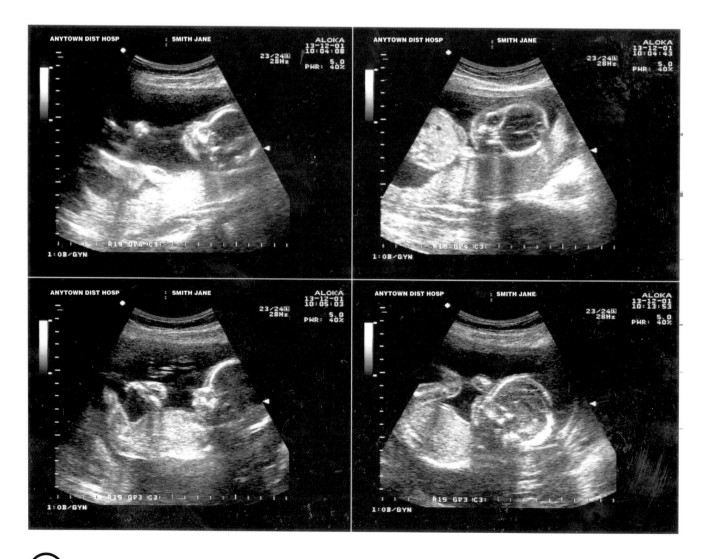

with the device producing the ultrasound waves, a special gel is applied to the region to be examined. This can be a bit cold but is completely harmless. It once took considerable training to interpret the pictures produced but they are now so clear the mum and dad can see for themselves. This can spoil the element of surprise when it come to the sex of the baby and you may be advised to 'look away' while the result is shown if you still want the mystery to remain.

Complications

So far as is known, ultrasound of the intensity and frequency used in scanning is completely harmless. Millions of pregnant women, and their babies, have had scans with no harm. You must balance the perception of danger from scanning against the consequences of an undetected serious malformation.

Uses of ultrasound

Without doubt the main advantage of routine ultrasound screening is the early detection and management of foetal abnormalities.

Ultrasound is extensively used in obstetrics mainly because of the possible danger of X-rays to the developing baby. Most pregnant women are screened at least once by ultrasound, usually around the 16 to 20th week of pregnancy. Ultrasound has many uses in maternity units. It can:

- Detect twins.
- Detect thickening of the neck tissues associated with Down's syndrome. This is called a nuchal scan.
- Display the position of the afterbirth (placenta). Problems arising from abnormal position, such as placenta praevia (where the placenta is blocking the 'way out' for the baby) can thus be managed.
- Facilitate amniocentesis, foetal blood sampling, chorionic villus sampling and foetoscopy.
- Confirm that the baby is of a size appropriate to the stage of pregnancy.
- Detect major foetal abnormalities such as anencephaly (poor brain development) and spina bifida (a lack of bone covering parts of the spinal cord).
- Measure the rates of blood flow through the heart valves and the large arteries of the baby's heart.
- Sometimes detect certain forms of congenital heart disease.
  Under ultrasound control, foetal blood samples can be obtained through a fine tube, and analysed to detect coagulation disorders, infections, haemoglobin abnormalities and immunodeficiency disorders.

Ultrasound enables the taking of biopsies (small samples of tissue). Blood transfusion in rhesus disease can be done while the baby is still in the womb, drug treatment given, and even certain forms of surgery can be performed guided by ultrasound.

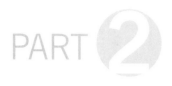
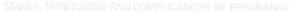
Chorionic villus sampling (CVS)

Introduction
CVS is similar to amniocentesis in that it involves collecting cells which are then examined to detect chromosomal abnormalities. The cells to be examined are taken from the placenta rather than from the amniotic fluid.

Which is better?
The main advantage of CVS over amniocentesis is that it can be performed earlier – typically between the 10th and 12th weeks of pregnancy – and the results are obtained more quickly. One disadvantage is that the test cannot detect spina bifida. CVS carries a small but significant risk of provoking a miscarriage, and the risk is slightly higher than with amniocentesis (0.5 to 1 per cent).

Neither amniocentesis nor CVS is performed without good reasons. These reasons may include the mother's age, the result of an earlier test or a family history of genetically-linked conditions. Which test is better will depend on the reasons for having it done and on the attitude of you and your partner to the risks associated with the test itself. These issues should be discussed with you before any decision is reached.

How it is performed
Depending on the doctor's preference and the position of the placenta, the cells may be obtained by passing a needle through the anaesthetised abdominal wall, or using a fine tube passed through the vagina and cervix.

What happens afterwards
Your partner will be told to take things easy for a few days and to watch for any signs of possible miscarriage.

Results are normally obtained within 3 or 4 days. Occasionally the cells taken for testing fail to grow in the laboratory and a repeat test is needed; this does not necessarily mean that there is anything wrong.

Again, any abnormal results will be explained to you by a specialist.

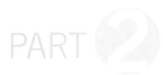

PART

Foetal heart monitoring

One of the best ways of telling whether the baby is in distress during labour is to monitor its heart beat. The 'low tech' method is to listen directly to the baby's heart with a simple form of stethoscope. Many men will have pre-empted this examination by the use of the cardboard liner of a toilet roll, which is a crude but effective way of listening to the baby.

This can be carried out electronically. One type of monitor is strapped to your partner's abdomen and the noise it produces has been used in many films. Once heard it is seldom forgotten. It also tends to have an hypnotic effect on conversation, producing lengthy silences as the baby's heart slows and accelerates with each contraction.

Alternatively, an electrode can be clipped to the scalp of the baby which gives a more accurate picture of what is happening and is less prone to stop during a large contraction, which just happens to be when you really want to know how the baby is getting on. The downside is that the mother-to-be will be less mobile with all these contraptions attached. It is possible to do this through telemetry (the same as with Formula 1 cars).

In some cases of distress where the heart of the baby is slowing and failing to recover quickly enough, blood may be taken from one of the small veins in the baby's scalp. It is an easy task to determine if there is sufficient oxygen present in the baby's blood or if it is being starved of its supply as it is being delivered.

There is a body of opinion that foetal heart monitoring gives rise to a high rate of interventions, such as caesarean section.

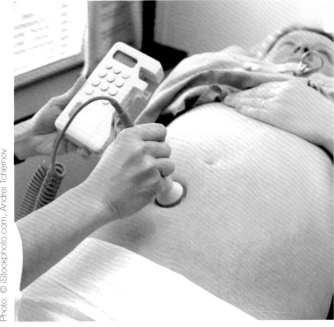

Photo: © iStockphoto.com, Andrei Tchernov

PART 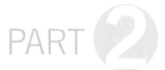 Spina bifida

Introduction

Neural tube defects, spina bifida, means that part of the spine is abnormally open so that the rear part of one or more of the vertebrae of the spine remain incomplete.

As a result, the spinal cord, which runs down through a series of holes in the vertebrae, can be unprotected in the affected area.

The severity of the defect varies considerably with many cases totally undiagnosed and causing no problem to the child or life as an adult. There are three levels: in spina bifida occulta, the condition is hidden and usually discoverable only on X-ray. In more serious cases, the coverings of the cord (the meninges) pass back through the opening to form a cyst-like swelling (a meningocele). In the most severe cases, the spinal cord itself is exposed. This is called a myelocele.

Symptoms

As with the severity of the defect the symptoms also vary widely. When there is a myelocele there is usually paralysis of the legs and loss of sensation. In more severe cases there may be total paralysis of the lower part of the body and incontinence. Repeated urinary tract infections may lead to kidney damage. An associated failure of normal circulation of the cerebrospinal fluid leads, in some cases, to 'water on the brain' (hydrocephalus).

Causes

As with many things in medicine we know what happens but not why. Spina bifida forms early in pregnancy when the spine is being formed. While the exact cause remains a mystery a lack of the vitamin folic acid early in pregnancy is a contributory factor.

Diagnosis

Ultrasound examination is often able to pick up the problem early in pregnancy giving the option of termination. Amniocentesis (see page 43) may also show a marked rise in the levels of alpha-fetoprotein in spina bifida.

Prevention

Myths abound, not least the discredited link with eating green potato. There is, however, good solid evidence that that a small daily intake of folic acid, taken before pregnancy and during early pregnancy, will substantially reduce the risk of spina bifida.

It is sufficient to take the vitamin for 28 days before conception and 12 weeks afterwards. No more than 0.4 mg per day is required for most women, which is well within the dose from commercial preparations available across the pharmacy counter, but to prevent a recurrence of a neural tube defect following one affected pregnancy a larger dose is required. To be most effective, folic acid must be being taken at an early stage of pregnancy as the spine is an early developmental feature.

Treatment

Surgery to correct the defect is usually performed as soon as possible after birth, but it may require further surgery later in life.

Folic acid substantially reduces the risk of spina bifida

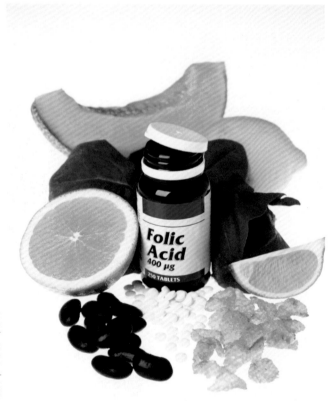

PART 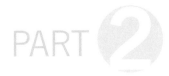 # Stillbirth

Introduction

Few disasters that life throws at you can compare with the birth of a dead baby. Often there is no obvious cause and you are left with a bewildering mix of emotions. It is confused with miscarriage but is said to occur after 24 weeks of pregnancy. The good news is that the number of stillbirths has fallen steadily during the last 50 years.

Causes

Some medical conditions increase the risk but often the reason will never be known:

- Diabetes.
- High blood pressure in the mother.
- Rhesus incompatibility (blue babies).
- Maternal high blood pressure and seizures in pregnancy (eclampsia).
- Severe malformations.
- Inadequacy of the afterbirth (placenta).
- Infections such as toxoplasmosis, German measles (rubella), syphilis or herpes simplex.

It is important to talk to your doctor about future babies as they can often give reassurance that this was a dreadful one-off and that it should not stop you from having a baby in future. On the other hand, they may be able to reduce the risk of it happening again by looking at any medical conditions that could have contributed.

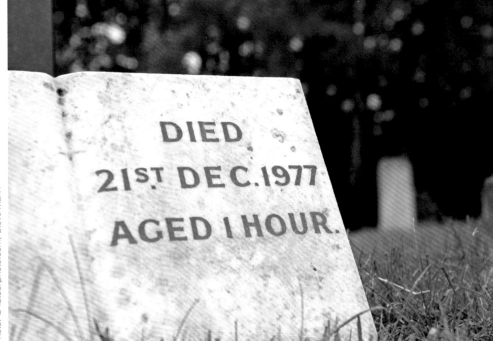

Photo: © iStockphoto.com, Steve Mann

PART 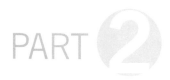 # Assisted delivery

Introduction

The reason why many doctors prefer hospital deliveries is that, unfortunately, not all deliveries go according to plan. Problems like a breech birth, where the bottom and not the head present first, however, can be predicted by good antenatal care including the use of ultrasound scans. Should a delivery pose a problem, if the second stage is too prolonged for instance, a number of alternatives can be used, depending on the nature of the problem.

Forceps & ventouse cup

Forceps conjure up all kinds of misconceptions. Not only can they save the life of the child but also avoid having to perform a caesarean section. They are essentially a pair of scoops which fit around the baby's head. Using gentle pulling, the doctor can manoeuvre the baby for a safe delivery. Despite all the old wives tales it is very safe when performed by an expert, although it does look a little dramatic. Ventouse cup is a vacuum-assisted delivery where a soft rubber cup is applied over the baby's head and a gentle suction applied which keeps the cup in place. the doctor can then manoeuvre the baby through its delivery. Both methods tend to cause some temporary distortion to the baby's head either from slight marks of the forceps, particularly about the ears, or a pronounced 'cap' on the baby's head from the vacuum delivery. Neither is permanent or dangerous. Again it is a balance of safety for the mother and child versus discomfort of the assisted delivery. Supporting your partner is important and many doctors will not only allow you stay with your partner but also prefer you do so.

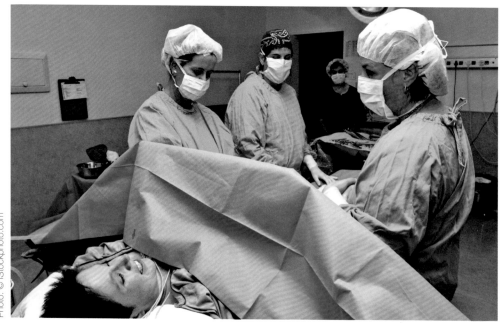

Photo: © iStockphoto.com

Caesarean section

Part of the reason why modern child birth is so much safer for the mother, is the speed at which the baby can be delivered by an operation should it prove impossible to allow a normal, or assisted, delivery. Placenta praevia, where the placenta is either over or very close to the opening of the womb, used to be fatal for both mother and child as there was no way of detecting its presence until delivery. Few women survived as there was invariably a great deal of blood loss. Thanks to ultrasound examination and caesarean section, this is now rarely the case.

The operation can be performed under a general anaesthetic or by 'freezing' the lower part of the body by injecting a local anaesthetic into the area around the lower spinal cord. This latter method allows the mother to see her baby as it is born and is pain free. You will be usually be invited to sit with your partner and is an experience which, like normal child birth, can be usefully shared. Be reassured that you will be protected from the nuts and bolts of the operation, allowing you to concentrate on supporting your partner. You will be surprised at the informality of the event, with every emphasis being made to allow you and your partner to enjoy your new baby.

Most babies will spend a little time in an incubator after a caesarean delivery as they can need a little more help keeping warm and getting enough air at the beginning.

Many women worry about the scar the operation will leave and the effect it could have on any future attempts at having children by a normal delivery. For almost all caesarean sections the scar will be very low down on the abdomen and run sideways, not up-and-down the abdomen. It is usually well covered by a pair of bikini bottoms and is often referred to as a 'bikini incision'.

While some complications of pregnancy and delivery which require a section may make a normal delivery dangerous, this is by no means true in all cases. It is your understanding of these points and help in the discussion which will reassure your partner when the day comes.

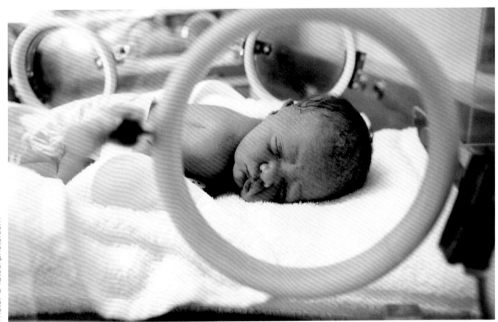

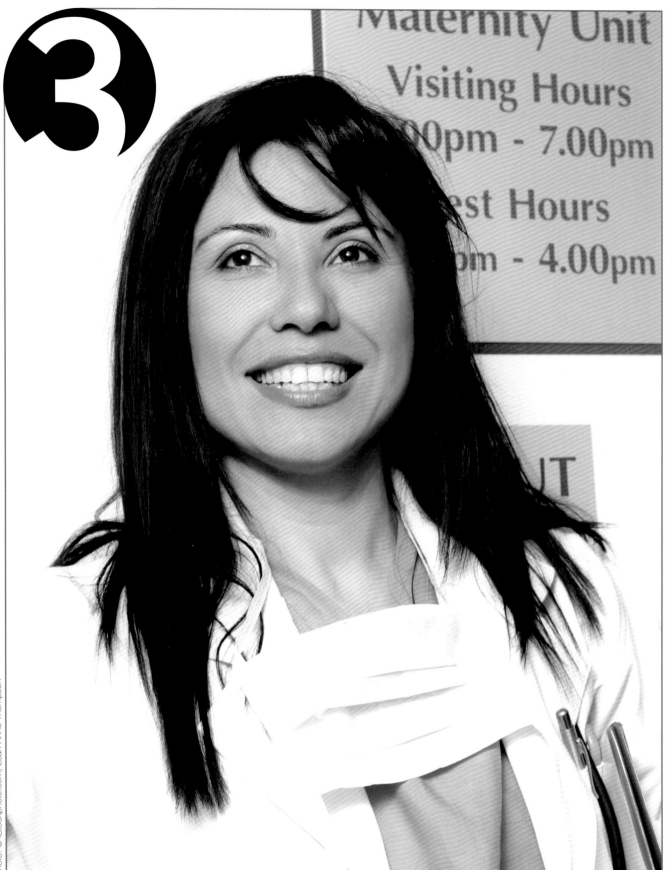

Maternity Unit
Visiting Hours
.00pm - 7.00pm
...est Hours
...m - 4.00pm

...IT

PART **3** # The birth and after

PART **3**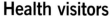

Health professionals

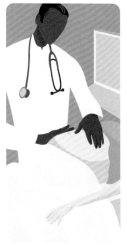

Introduction

Let's face it, health professionals all look alike. Once you could tell who was the doctor by the stethoscope in their white coat pocket. Now they all run around with theatre greens on like ER. Their name badge should be a giveaway, but don't be afraid to ask who they are and what they do.

Health visitors

Nurses with extra training for caring in the community. Although they will take a special interest in your baby they look after the whole family. Generally they will visit about 10 days after the baby is born and check whether you or your partner have any problems or need any help. They are not always based at the doctor's surgery, you may need to contact the health centre.

General practitioners

GPs are often involved in antenatal shared care. Few are prepared to deliver at home, but may do deliveries in community hospitals.

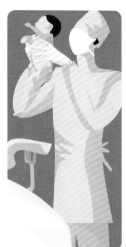

Obstetricians

These are doctors specialising in pregnancy, labour and often gynaecology. Most women will see the consultant infrequently during antenatal care unless there is a particular reason for doing so. Most complicated deliveries are performed by obstetricians. If you or your partner are concerned you can ask to see them during your antenatal visit or book in for the next one.

Paediatricians

These doctors are generally on hand during a complicated birth or a caesarean section. They will check the baby shortly after birth to make sure all is well, and are the person to talk through any concerns over the baby.

Midwives

Predominately but not exclusively female, they will deliver most babies and perform most antenatal checks. They can work either in hospital or in the community, or sometimes work in both environments.

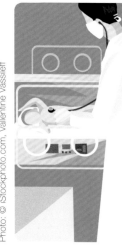

Anaesthetists

All anaesthetics, whether general or spinal, are performed by anaesthetists. You can talk to them about the most appropriate form of pain relief during labour.

Genetic counsellors

Doctors, nurses and scientists all work in the area of advice on genetic problems. If there is a family history of a congenital condition you can discuss the likelihood of this affecting your baby.

Photo: © iStockphoto.com, Vallentine Vassileff

PART 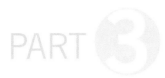 **Changing GP/midwife**

Introduction

Working with your health professionals is the key to better care. Getting the best from them is a team effort but if things are not going well you need to know how to upgrade to better performance.

Never underestimate the value of a good midwife or GP. They will support you when things are bad, give encouragement when it's needed but also recognise your own abilities and common sense. Even so, sometimes you and your health professional just don't get along. If you feel that a poor relationship is having an impact on your care, then you do have the right to find someone else to look after you. Changing your GP, midwife or health visitor can be a challenge, but while it is not something you would want to do every day, it is not too difficult when you do have to make a change.

Changing your GP

The vast majority of changes for people's GPs are because of changing house; we are a very mobile population compared to 30 years ago. If you are simply moving house, all you need to do is apply to a GP in your new area.

Being unhappy with your GP is a different matter, and although it is possible to change without giving a reason it is better to send a letter or explain in person so that any problems can be addressed in future. Most problems with GPs result from pressure of work and communication misunderstandings.

Your health authority has to find you an alternative GP, or send you details of how to change and a list of doctors. They must do so within two working days. Once you have changed, they should send any records needed urgently and transfer remaining records within six weeks.

At the same time, doctors also have to right to remove you from their list without giving a reason for doing so, although most will at least try to explain why they are taking this drastic action. Your health authority must make sure you are not left without a doctor.

There is nothing wrong with asking advice from a number of sources. For instance, you can remain with your original doctor but consult with another on contraceptive and maternity issues, if you choose. Contact your health authority to find out which doctors have a 'C' after their name for contraceptive issues and contact the same place for maternity issues asking which doctors are on the 'obstetric list'.

Changing your midwife

Changing your partner's midwife depends on how she was originally assigned her midwife in the first place. There are no tablets of stone and although you and your partner may have been assigned a midwife early on you can ask for a change at any point. You and your partner may receive all your maternity care from the hospital. In this case, if you have an objection to

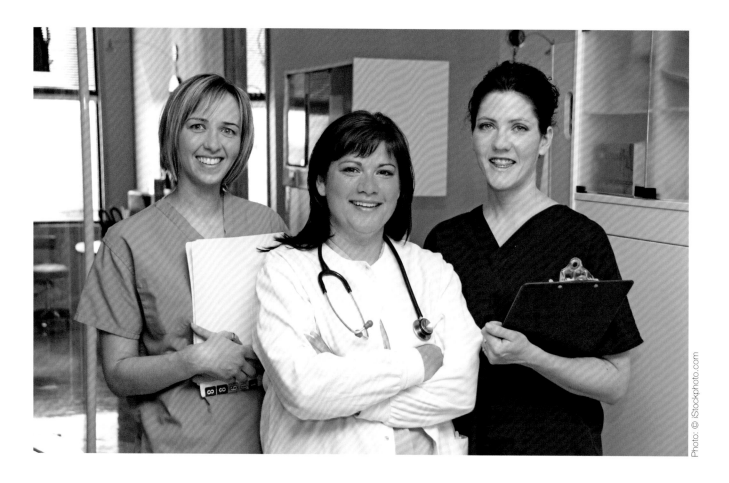

a particular midwife then raise your problem with the Head of Midwifery Services. He or she will listen to your problem and if they feel it is valid, try to arrange an alternative midwife. Caution is advised. Knowing each other and having insight into any potential problem is valuable. In truth, given the pressure on the NHS, you may find that hospital care means a different midwife on nearly every visit, so it may be less of a problem.

Shared care between a hospital and GP also tends to mean your partner will see a number of midwives, at least on their hospital visits. Requesting a different midwife at hospital is done in the same way as above. A different midwife at your GP may be more of a problem as midwives are usually 'assigned' to a practice. She may have to go elsewhere for her care if she doesn't want to be treated by a certain midwife.

The final type of care is entirely from a midwife, as part of a team of midwives. In this case your partner is usually assigned two midwives who carry out nearly all your partner's care, including delivery. You and your partner could request to be moved to another team of two if you felt strongly about one midwife. Again, the Health of Midwifery Services will be able to give you guidance.

PART 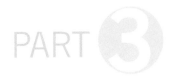 **Appointments**

Introduction

Huge amounts of GP, midwife and practice nurse appointments are lost each year simply because appointments are missed. This means that it takes longer to get an appointment and valuable appointment time is wasted.

You can help by making sure that you either keep your appointment or cancel it.

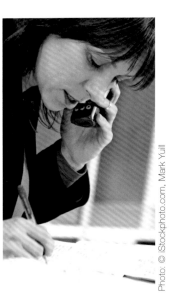

Photo: © iStockphoto.com, Mark Yuill

What do appointments cost?

It has been calculated that each daytime appointment with a GP costs £20.

Even though you do not pay directly for an appointment it is a waste of NHS resources if the appointment is missed.

When is it too late to cancel?

The earlier you cancel the appointment the better – but it's never too late to cancel, provided you do so before the start time of the appointment.

What if I can't make it?

Cancel the appointment! Call your surgery to cancel it as soon as possible. If you can't get through the first time, please don't give up.

If you get through to an answer machine please leave a message stating:
- Your name.
- Your appointment time and date.
- Who your appointment is with.

Don't forget it

We all forget things sometimes – don't forget your health. A common reason for missing appointments is that people forget. Here are some useful tips to help you remember:
- Make a note of your appointment as soon as you book it and stick this card somewhere obvious like a notice board.
- If you have a mobile phone, why not set the alarm beforehand?
- If you have a diary or note book write in the time and date straight away.
- Have your GP surgery number saved in your mobile or written down with your other numbers.
- If you tend to be forgetful let someone like a partner, family member, carer or colleague know so they can remind you.
- Stick a Post-it note somewhere obvious like on your fridge, phone or computer.
- If your appointment is during work time, make sure it is at a convenient time, double check with your boss that it is ok to get time off and give yourself plenty of time to get to the surgery.
- Most importantly, don't put off seeing the GP if you need to. The earlier you get help the better for your health.

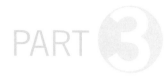

PART

Antenatal care & pain relief

Introduction

Your partner will be offered a choice of ways she can have antenatal care. This will be influenced by her previous pregnancies, medical health and social factors such as living in a remote part of the country. Being pregnant is not an illness. Having babies is undoubtedly painful and may occasionally be a tad tricky but it is still normal and women have been doing it for a very long time.

Hospital-based care

Women in their first pregnancy, where there is some reason to want closer observation or if there were some problems with a previous pregnancy, are often advised full hospital care. A named consultant and a named midwife will take responsibility for your partner's checks as she approaches her delivery date. Parental classes are usually held in the same department and men are made very welcome.

During ultrasound scans it is easy to underestimate how scared your partner can be at that first session. A hot sweaty hand in her hotter sweatier hand helps more than you will know.

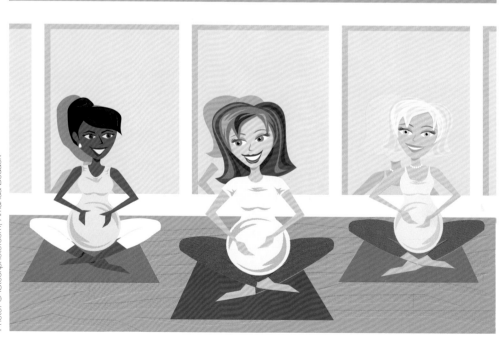

Photo: © iStockphoto.com, Amanda Bodack

It's easy to forget in that darkened room with the glowing totally incomprehensible screen that abnormalities are rare and all unusual positions in the womb can be safely dealt with. Mention of 'Alien: Now this is personal' is never appreciated!

Shared care

Most GPs will offer a mix of checks at their surgery along with visits to the maternity hospital. Convenient and quick, it also ensures contact with a doctor who generally knows a lot about your partner's medical history. You can also attend these, just like the hospital sessions.

Tests

There are routine checks made for simple things like anaemia, diabetes and blood groups, but infections which can harm the baby are also checked with your partner's consent. HIV is not routinely tested for unless you ask. Times change and so does treatment. Modern medicines have extended life span considerably. We know an awful lot more about pregnancy and HIV as well, but it is useless if nobody knows whether HIV is involved.

Other tests check for sickle cell disease in Black Afro Caribbean people and thalassaemia in people with Mediterranean or Asian origins, both of which can affect babies even though there is no evidence of either condition in the parents. Tests can predict the chances of this happening, allowing you to make decisions early on.

Pain relief

No matter how much women and men know about childbirth there is always the 'what if' factor to contend with. Pain is one of the greatest fears, for both partners. There are choices of pain relief from a complete absence of pain to no interference

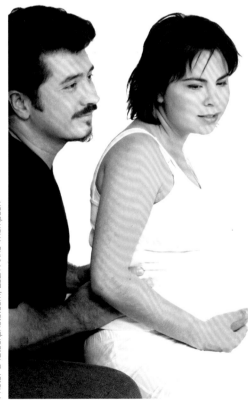

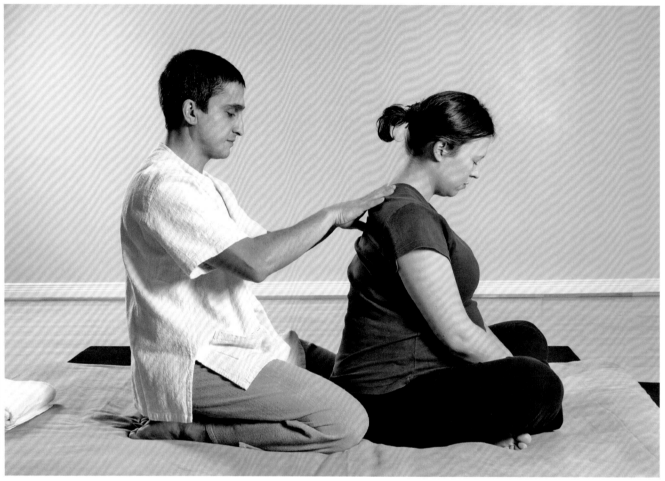

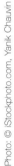

at all. Each extreme has its own advantage, zero pain can mean immobility during an epidural while some women want to experience childbirth in its entirety without any pain relief. Most important to remember and get through to your partner is that it will end. Most pain is endurable so long as there is definitely an end to it. This made easier by having someone there whom they trust to tell them it is worth it, that something good will come from it and that there is an incredible thing happening which is far better to focus on than the pain.

Whatever path she chooses you can supply the distraction, cool towel on the head, back rubbing and most of all, encouragement. Some people say men don't belong at the delivery. Possibly, but it's up to you two, not the midwife or doctor. It's your baby. It's worth remembering that pain was once thought to be an essential part of childbirth and requests for relief considered to be ungodly.

Entonox (gas and air)
Your partner will have control over the amount of gas she breaths by holding the mask herself. It works best if inhaled

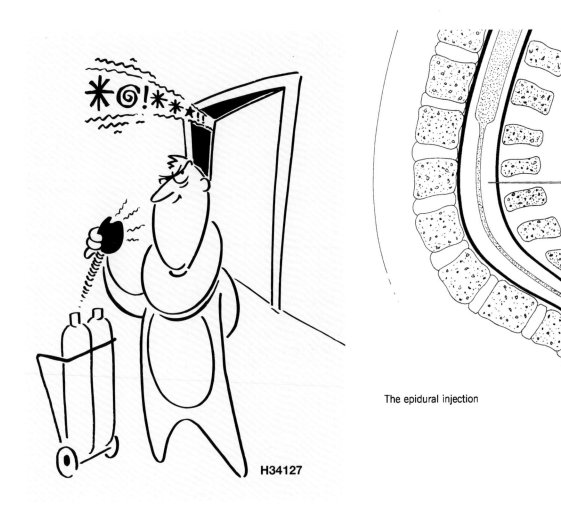

H34127

The epidural injection

H34111

just before each contraction, so check yourself by keeping your hand on her bump and gently warning her to start sucking as you feel the contractions start. Entonox is safe for both mum and baby but does tend to abolish any lady-like notions about bad language. Brace yourself for some toe curling oaths. It can cause drowsiness; relaying instructions from the midwife or doctor is your job as she will often hear no one else's voice. No matter how much noise she is making you don't need to shout. Keep your voice calm, she will still hear you.

Pethidine

Although pethidine is highly effective it can only be used at certain stages of labour as it affects the baby's ability to breathe properly if given too late. An antidote is sometimes given to the baby if this happens. It can also cause severe nausea.

Epidurals

Tiny amounts of anaesthetic injected around the lower part of the spine have miraculous effect on pain during childbirth. Unfortunately it is difficult for the mum to sense what is happening and she must rely even more on the instructions from the team. It also blocks any sensation, let alone movement, in her legs, which can persist after the baby is born.

Things you should know and expect with epidurals:

- They are safe but look scary.
- She will be paralysed, not just pain free, from the waist down. On its own this is scary. Try rubbing and massaging her legs.
- An intense headache affects around 1 in 250 women and a sudden drop in blood pressure is fairly common. She will feel faint and sick at first but it will pass. Reassurance really does help.
- Sensation returns like the dreaded pins and needles of frozen hands. Massage her legs while she gives the cause of all this misery hugs and kisses.

Other methods

There are other methods of pain relief including electrical blockage of pain signals (TENS) and hypnosis. Talk it through with someone who has tried them first.

PART

The Big Push (labour & childbirth)

Introduction

Labour wards are designed, obviously, for labouring women not expectant fathers. Even though the mother must fast for sound medical reasons, it makes sense to have a partner who is not about to collapse from hunger during a long delivery. Simply providing some form of basic refreshment will help you during delivery.

Education and preparation for the expectant father are both helpful and important, but most of us have absolutely no idea of the emotional upheaval we are about to live through. Many men feel like a 'spare part' yet the impact the presence of a partner can have on the confidence of a woman about to give birth cannot be understated. Men have a role to play, and with greater insight into the way a baby is born, a man can not only experience the miracle of birth but also make an invaluable contribution. This bit helps provide that insight.

Planning ahead

Time off work is not guaranteed for a father in all countries. Early or late deliveries can put all the best-laid plans to naught. Two weeks past the 'expected date of delivery' is not unusual but can cause a disproportionate amount of confusion and worry.

Work out beforehand how you will get to the hospital. This is particularly important as labour can start at any time. If you do not have a car and cannot depend upon relatives or neighbours, call an ambulance explaining what is happening.

Labour wards tend to be very hot places. Go prepared for the heat - wear shorts and a tee shirt, and take some bottled water.

Make sure you have the means of telephoning relatives - coins, phone cards or enough credit on the mobile phone, plus of course a list of phone numbers.

As the day draws near, keep a bag packed with the things you will need. Your partner will have her own list and her own bag (or bags). Your bag should contain survival items for you and treats for you both. And don't forget the camera!

Labour

Although most women are quite certain when labour has started, it is easy to mistake other things happening for the onset of labour. First pregnancies are a time for some confusion over contractions which may have little to do with labour.

The uterus contracts about every fifteen to twenty minutes during pregnancy and these contractions last around twenty to thirty seconds. Such contractions are felt as a tightening around the abdomen. These 'Braxton-Hicks' contractions become more frequent and stronger towards the end of pregnancy and can be confused with the onset of true labour. The Braxton-Hicks

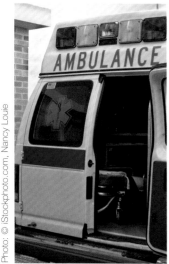

Induction of labour

Inducing labour was introduced in 1969 as a means of reducing the number of prolonged labours. Its aim was to keep labour to less than 12 hours and assisted delivery (eg, forceps) rates to a minimum. It was originally designed for starting labour in first-time pregnancies with a single baby. It has been modified significantly over time, but the core principles remain:

- Early diagnosis of the need to induce labour, following strict criteria, by a senior midwife.
- Checking for dilating rate by vaginal examination hourly for 3 hours then every 2 hours, at least.
- Amniotomy (rupturing the membrane around the sac containing the baby) 1 hour after admission.
- If not dilating at rate of 1 cm/hour a drug is given to increase the rate of dilation.
- Women not in labour should be sent home although 50% are readmitted within 24 hours.
- Personal, psychological support for the woman.
- Proactive use of epidural anaesthesia (see page 61) on demand from the mother.
- Regular checks by the obstetrician.
- Regularly checking the way the process within the obstetric unit was working and any problems it might be causing.

At the end of the day, and it often is, induction of labour should be used only when it is thought that the baby will be safer in the outside world than in the womb. The National Institute for Clinical Excellence (NICE) guidelines clearly defined its use in clinical practice.

- It should be offered to women with healthy pregnancy after 41 weeks as the risk of stillbirth roughly doubles with each week over term.
- It should be offered before term to women whose pregnancy is complicated by diabetes.
- In women whose waters have broken (the sac has ruptured prematurely) after 37 weeks which happens in around 6 to 19% of pregnancies. They should be given a choice of different levels of induction.

Commonest reasons for inducing labour are:

- Prolonged pregnancy – 70% of such cases are induced after 41 weeks often at the mother's request. Obstetrician will usually agree if the cervix is ready.
- Suspected baby growth retardation.
- Hypertension and eclampsia – approximately 50% women with this problem are induced.
- Planned time of delivery in best interests of baby, eg, cardiac abnormalities may need immediate surgery after birth.

Induction procedure

The commonest method of induction in UK is placing prostaglandin gel or pessary high in the vagina. The drug is absorbed through the vaginal and cervical skin. There must be regular checks by the midwife or obstetrician.

Complications

Possible complications of induction include those of normal delivery not least that a caesarean section may be required. On top of these are:

- Too rapid stimulation of contractions causing foetal distress and possible lack of oxygen to the baby.
- Rupture of the womb especially in women with more than one previous birth.
- Intrauterine infection with prolonged membrane rupture without delivery (less likely if labour occurs within 12 hours).
- Possible prolapsed cord (where the cord comes out first) can occur with first rush of amniotic fluid.
- Amniotic fluid embolism where the fluid gets into the blood stream of the mother casing a blockage.
- 1.5 times the risk of forceps vaginal delivery and 1.8 times the risk of caesarean section.

This all sounds very stark but child birth is infinitely safer than ever before. Even so there are those who feel that some doctors intervene far too soon for reasons not necessarily in the best interest of mother and child. By understanding the reasons for inducing labour it will be easier for your partner to make a decision she is most happy with.

What you can do

- Support her in her decision. 'Always knew it was a bad idea from the outset' never goes down well.
- Recognise that she will be fully aware this is not 'normal' and so may be more scared especially if it is her first birth.
- Reassure her constantly, but keep your mind open to potential problems developing. You know her better than any of the delivery team. Communicate concerns to them as clearly and calmly as you can.
- Respect her requests for privacy during the procedure. It will be your joint decision as to whether you should be there for the start of the procedure.
- Monitoring equipment is more commonly used during induction, and the equipment and the noises it makes can be intimidating and even frightening. Distraction is better than obsessively following each blip of the baby's heart rate.
- Keep at the back of your mind that there was a reason for induction and this may change things later on. A tad greater fuss being made over the baby is routine and doesn't mean things have gone horribly wrong.
- Holding her hand and cold towels on her forehead will do wonders.

contractions become more frequent in the third trimester and all the symptoms worsen due to a growing increase in pressure within the abdomen.

If there is doubt, you should ring your doctor or midwife and be prepared to answer the following questions:
● How long have the contractions been present?
● At what intervals are they occurring?
● How long do they last?
● Has there been a 'show' (a watery, mucus discharge, often tinged with blood, from the vagina)?

If the labour is really taking place, the contractions will have been present for some time, even hours. Usually the interval between each contraction will be less than twenty minutes and the duration will be more than forty seconds.

Your partner should not eat before going in to hospital, as the administration of a general anaesthetic, should it be needed, can be dangerous with food present in the stomach.

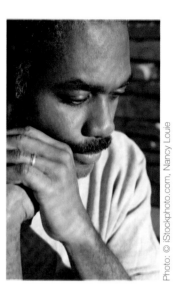

Photo: © iStockphoto.com, Nancy Louie

The real thing

Ritual still lives in childbirth, even in our supposedly advanced society. Thankfully we no longer shave the pubic hair and fathers are welcome in most labour wards. But in ritual is a form of safety in familiarity. Breaking the ritual can be seen as 'bad luck'. Mercifully few of the rules of the labour ward have more to do with this form of protection than sound clinical practice. Treating the father as a useless lump of dad, prone to trip over the drip or switch off the heart monitor instead of the TV, however, is a waste of valuable resource. Having a job to do, such as masseur, water-bearer or a source of moral support is infinitely better than wearing out the carpet in the waiting room. Worse still, dads can be ignored, as if they are some sort of wall-hanging. Few men will have the pleasure of delivering their own child, but the support and love they give to their partner during childbirth is part of the bonding process which is often applied only to the mother.

Premature delivery can be postponed using certain drugs for a while particularly if the baby is not yet developed enough to have a reasonable chance of survival. There is also a dangerous period before 40 weeks where the baby's lungs are most at risk from poor function due to the lack of a lubricating protein which keeps the tubes open. Most obstetricians would want at least 36 weeks but some babies will survive even earlier. There are basically three stages of labour.

Stages of labour

These overlap and vary in time, often considerably, from woman to woman.

The first stage

After the membrane which surrounds the baby ruptures it releases the liquid in which the baby floats. Breaking of the waters, as it is known, can produce a varying amount of fluid. Some women can confuse this with simply passing water, particularly if there are no contractions at the time. Usually, however, the membranes will not rupture until well into labour. This first stage of labour continues until the cervix, the neck of the womb, is fully dilated. During this time the position of the baby will be determined. This may involve an internal examination to check the progress of labour and to assess the position of the baby's head. Most babies are born head first, rather than in the breech, or head following, position.

The second stage
During the second stage of labour the baby's head appears, usually face down and rotates either way until facing to one or other side. Obviously it is important that this stage does not take too long but equally it has to be slow enough not to cause damage as the baby's head passes through the small confines of the birth canal in the pelvis. Your partner will want to push very hard at this point and it is important that you relay to her all the instructions from the midwife. You are aiming for a steady controlled appearance of the baby's head rather than like a champagne cork being popped. Simply talking to her and giving encouragement is enough, although a cool wet cloth on her forehead along with helping with the gas mixture, makes her job a little easier. She may well use language that you never heard her say before. Equally, many women will shout at the people trying to help. Importantly, many women say that the only voice they could hear during this stage of labour was that of their partner. It is easy to understand this given the effects of the pain, anxiety and any drugs given to ease the pain.

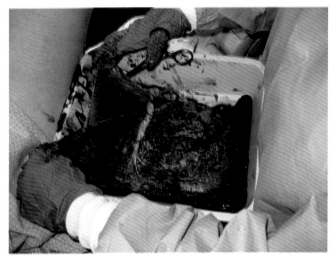

The afterbirth (placenta)

If the second stage of labour is unduly prolonged, or if certain problems develop, the care team may decide that some assistance is required. This can mean using a ventouse (suction) cup or forceps to help the birth, or a caesarean section. See *Assisted Delivery* on page 50

To prevent any severe tearing of the vagina, the midwife may perform an episiotomy which involves cutting the lower part of the vaginal wall as the baby's head is appearing. Local anaesthetic is always applied first but it still looks barbaric. After a short while following the birth this will be repaired by stitching. It helps if you are there to help maintain the distraction and provide support.

The third stage
The third stage of labour involves the passing of the afterbirth. It is a surprisingly large organ and is always examined carefully by the midwife to check that all of it has been passed.

Mystery has always surrounded the placenta and probably with good reason. It is responsible for allowing the exchange of oxygen and waste gases between mother and baby. It allows the free passage of vital foods and vitamins but stops most pathogens (organisms) which would harm the baby. Even the mother's own blood is not allowed to cross the placental barrier. The placenta sorts out what is needed by the baby and what is harmful. It is made up of a mixture cells from the baby and those from the mother. When it is understood that the baby is actually a 'foreign body' as far as the mother is concerned, and yet the baby is not normally attacked by the mother's defence system, it gives some insight into the sophistication of the placenta. At times this balance is broken down and the baby is aborted by the mother's immune system. Similarly the cells of the placenta may make an uncontrolled invasion of the mother and actually cause a rare form of cancer, now thankfully treatable.

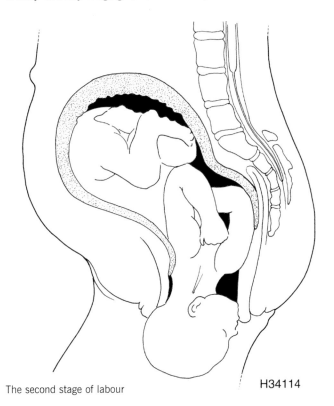

The second stage of labour

H34114

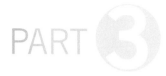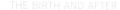

PART **3**

New baby

First impressions

Newly born babies are always short of air as they are born so they invariably appear blue. This is completely normal, as is the fine white cheesy substance (vernix) which covers their bodies. Most babies' faces look distorted along with their heads. Remember that the head has to mould itself in order to get through the narrow canal. A few good breaths, a quick rub and they actually look almost human.

Not all babies cry when they are born, although it is encouraging if they do as it means they are expanding their lungs which have also been squeezed during birth. Both the squeezing and the crying help to get rid of the fluid which is always present in their lungs. Most adults, including men, on the other hand, weep unashamedly. Few men, no matter how big or tough, can resist this little bundle when handed to them.

Relief is usually the first emotion, closely followed by awe at the presence of new life. Most men talk of their admiration for their partner, but it is difficult to put into words the emotion felt by any father at the birth of their child. Bonding is said to take place between baby and mother; a similar process takes place not only between father and baby but between man and woman. Furthermore, this extension of love encompasses much of the family, and is undiluted by the number of children a man may have.

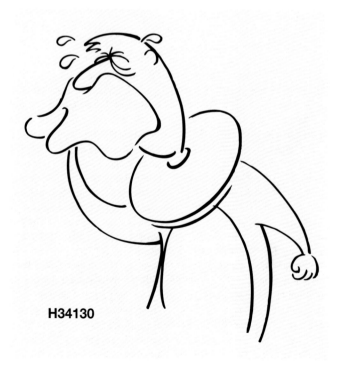

H34130

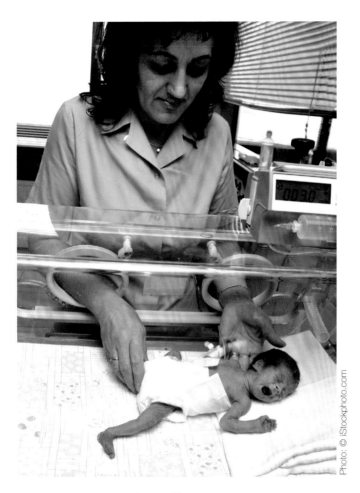

Photo: © iStockphoto.com

Incubators and jaundice

Seeing your baby in an incubator for the first time can be distressing. Even more so for the mother. Such is the caution of modern medicine that the baby is given every assistance possible in the vital early hours and days of birth. In most cases it is a short-term aid, often in response to 'Apgar' scores which are lower than optimal (see page 188). As the baby is born, the midwife or doctor will assess your baby for such things as muscle tone, the speed of breathing, heart rate and colour. This is checked again a short time afterwards and the results are combined as a score. Just because your baby is placed in an incubator does not mean there is a serious problem.

Temperature regulation is poor at the beginning and breathing may be laboured. An incubator supplies assistance for both. It is, however, a physical barrier and can inhibit the natural bonding which occurs particularly between mother and child. Most hospitals now encourage, whenever possible, the mother and father to handle the baby while in the incubator. If needed, drips will be used to supply fluid if your baby is having difficulty with breathing. This is particularly distressing for parents.

If jaundice, which is also very common after delivery, should reach levels which might interfere with the baby's brain, ultra violet lights are used to help break down the pigment which causes the colouration in the skin. Now that the blood type of the baby can be predicted and rhesus incompatibility be avoided, blood exchanges for 'blue babies' where the mother's immune system destroys the blood of the baby, has become uncommon.

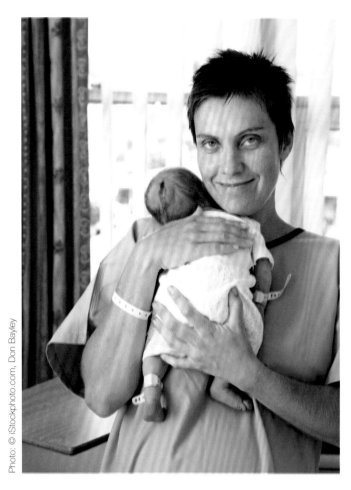

After care

Most maternity units now favour having the mother up and about as soon as possible after delivery, even following a caesarean section. Similarly they tend to go home much sooner than previously. For mothers this is a time of excitement and fulfilment, bringing home a new baby. Relatives and well-wishers will congregate en masse. Some will say 'Well I know she has had a lot of visitors, but I know she would want to see me'. There is a happy balance between having a few adoring people round and turning it into a circus. Gentle persuasion down the telephone advising a postponed visit can help.

Fear of the unknown

Death of a child during birth is not usually contemplated by the father to any great extent. Loss of their partner is even further from their minds. Such is power of modern expectation in contemporary medicine. More likely a dad will be worried about the pain and distress of their partner and the fear of a malformed baby.

Disappointment of the desired sex of the child will come after the confirmation of normality. This fear is highest for the first birth and worse for any birth after a previously-affected child.

Hidden emotion

Being male has many advantages, not least that you are the one who only has to say push. It is not all on the plus side, however, and many men will find it difficult to cry in public. Holding a baby is natural, and men, despite their concern for dropping the new baby, catch on very quickly. It is rare for the man to have the first cuddle except following a caesarean section by general anaesthetic.

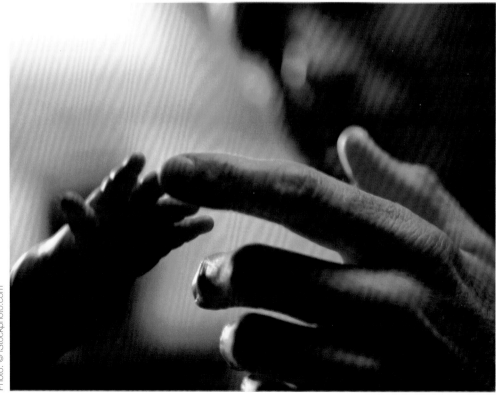

PART 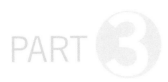 Circumcision

Introduction

Circumcision goes back into distant history and was a part of the initiation ritual for many cultures. Opinions on the medical and social merits of circumcision have been debated for years. Although less than 4 per cent of British boys are medically circumcised, some experts consider that this is still far too many. Medically, the real incidence of cases actually requiring the operation is said to be less than 1 per cent.

As the foreskin is quite firmly attached to the bulb (glans) of the penis during the first few years of life it is normal not to be able to retract it and should not be a justification for circumcision. The opening at the tip of the foreskin is normally quite small and will stretch in time. The foreskin should not be pulled back in infancy but occasional attempts at gentle retraction will do no harm to small boys and will help to stretch the skin.

Later, it is important that the foreskin should be retracted so that smegma which collects under it can be washed away every day, although there is no clear evidence that it causes cancer of the penis or cervical cancer in women, as once thought. There is some evidence however, that circumcision can reduce the chances of infection from HIV.

Why it is necessary

Although circumcision is rarely necessary for medical reasons, in a small number of boy babies the opening in the foreskin is so small that urine can't be released easily. This can cause ballooning of the foreskin when the baby is urinating and is called is called phimosis. Debate ensues over the possibility of this causing kidney problems in later life and some paediatricians might consider circumcision.

How it is performed

The operation is performed either under a local anaesthetic injection injected around the base of the penis and into the base of the foreskin, or under a general anaesthetic for older children. Why it should be thought that a very young baby feels less pain is a mystery to many.

Recovery

Unless performed by non-medically qualified surgeons, complications are uncommon. Infection and scar tissue are the main complications. Some men seek to re-grow their foreskin later in life and although this requires great perseverance, it can be done by using a stretching technique.

Circumcision is rarely needed for medical reasons

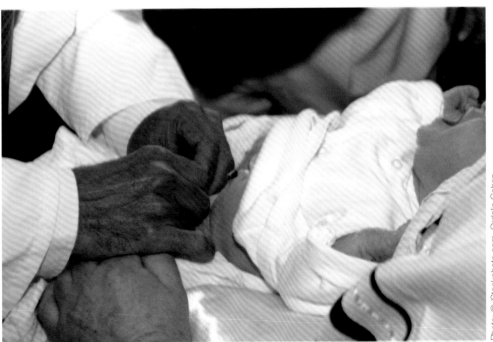

Photo: © iStockphoto.com, Ordelia Cohen

PART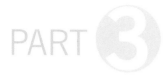

Immunisation

Childhood immunisation is one of the main reasons we have eradicated many childhood diseases in this country. By boosting your child's immune response they can fight infections which once killed or maimed countless millions of children. Polio is now history and measles no longer infects children in the USA. The EU aims to eradicate measles and rubella (German Measles) within the next decade or so. Some children will be left less protected because they:

● Cannot be immunised for medical reasons.
● Cannot get to the vaccine services.
● Are one of the few where the vaccine doesn't work.

If enough children are vaccinated this will not matter as the 'herd' immunity will prevent the spread of infection.

Even the so-called common childhood conditions such as whooping cough can kill. It is therefore very important to protect children from these diseases.

Despite much media attention there is still no definite link proven between the triple vaccine MMR with either Crohn's disease or autism. Using the vaccine separately is possible but is less effective than the combined injection and does, of course, triple the number of injections required for full protection. In

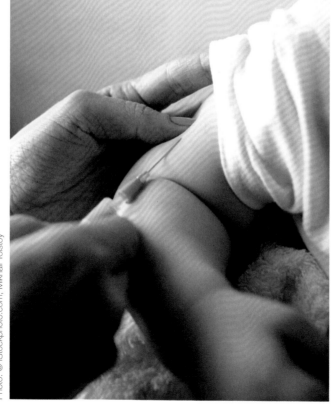

Photo: © iStockphoto.com, Mikhail Tolstoy

those countries where the MMR uptake has declined there has been a corresponding increase in the number of measles cases. If you are concerned about having your child immunised, contact your health visitor to discuss your concerns.

Serious reactions to the vaccination are rare but inflammation and itchness at the injections site is common as is a temporary fever. Baby preparations of paracetamol or ibuprofen can help (always read the label first).

If you miss a vaccination appointment, you do not have to start the course of vaccines again. The recommended gap between vaccines is an ideal – if you miss one, just make a new appointment as soon as you can.

The following is a guide to the recommended timetable for immunisations.

Age	Immunisation (vaccine given)
2 months	**DTP/Polio/Hib** (Diphtheria, Tetanus, Pertussis, Polio, and Haemophilus Influenza B) all in one injection, plus: **Pneumococcal (PCV)** in a separate injection
3 months	**DTP/Polio/Hib** (2nd dose), plus: **MenC (Meningococcus Group C)** in a separate injection
4 months	**DTP/Polio/Hib** (3rd dose), plus: **MenC** (2nd dose) in a separate injection, plus: **Pneumococcal (PCV)** (2nd dose) in a separate injection
Around 12 months	**Hib/MenC** (combined as one injection - 4th dose of Hib and 3rd dose of MenC)
Around 13 months	**MMR** (Measles, Mumps and Rubella combined as one injection), plus: **Pneumococcal (PCV)** (3rd dose) in a separate injection
Around 4-5 years	'Pre-school' booster of **DTP/Polio**, plus: **MMR** (second dose) in a separate injection
Around 13-18 years	**Td/Polio** booster. (A combined injection of Tetanus, low dose Diphtheria, and Polio.)
Adults	**Influenza and Pneumococcal** if you are aged 65 or over **Td/Polio** - at any age if you were not fully immunised as a child

Note

DTP, Polio and Hib vaccines are combined into one injection - the DTP/Polio/Hib vaccine.

Pneumococcal (PCV) is a separate injection and was added to the routine immunisation schedule in September 2006.

Meningococcus group C vaccine (MenC) is sometimes given as a separate injection but is combined with Hib for one injection.

Td/Polio is Tetanus, low dose Diphtheria and Polio vaccines combined as one injection.

Polio immunisation changed in 2004. The polio vaccine is now combined with DPT/Hib or Td and given by injection. It used to be given by mouth (oral vaccine) as a few drops of vaccine on the tongue. If you have previously started a course of polio immunisation with oral vaccine you can finish off the course with polio injections. You do not need to start again.

Measles, mumps and rubella vaccines are combined into one injection - the MMR vaccine.

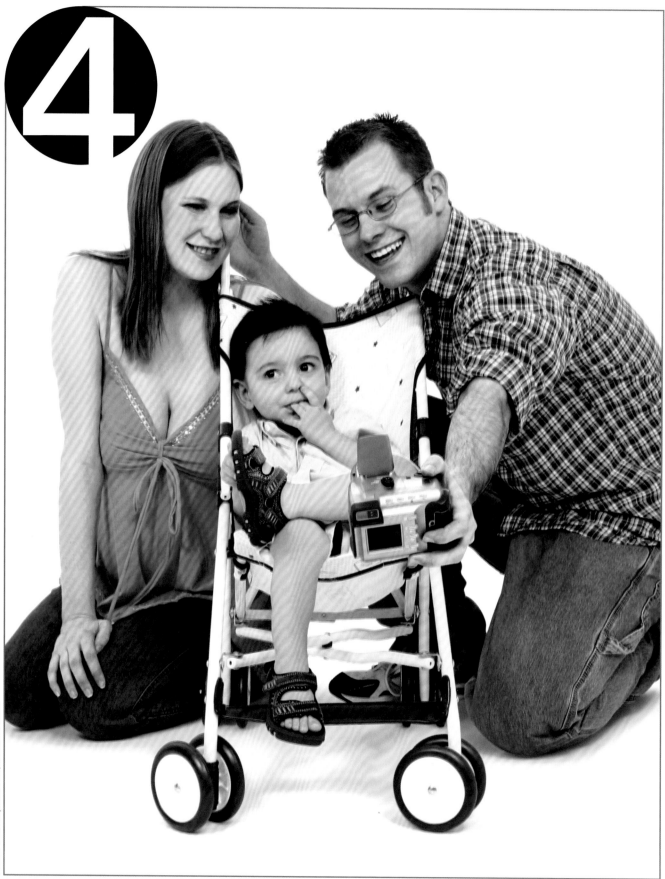

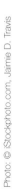

PART **4** BABY MANUAL

New routine

PART 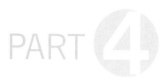 **Life goes on**

Introduction

Less than half of all childcare is carried out by fathers, mainly because poor flexibility at work prevents them from doing more. On average, dads of under five year olds devote about three and a half hours a day to childcare – an improvement from a mere quarter of an hour per day in the mid 1970s. (Equal Opportunities Commission 'Shared caring: bringing fathers into the frame' 2005).

A total of 80 per cent of fathers and 85 per cent of mothers, compared to only 62 per cent of employers, believe everyone should be able to balance their work and home lives in the way they want. Nearly two fifths of dads work over 48 hours a week and one in eight clocks up over 60 hours. Satisfaction with work-life balance was, not surprisingly, found to be much lower in those working longer. Despite many employers saying work-life balance practices helped foster good employment relations, more than half of all those surveyed didn't offer any form of flexible working and less than 10 per cent offered crèche facilities. This has the knock-on effect for women of limiting their choice over work and family commitment. If nothing else this tells us that child care can take two to tango. It also says much about the value of planning for children rather than having surprises pop up every nine months or so.

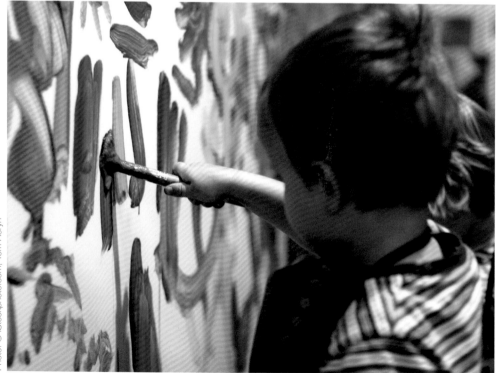

Photo: © iStockphoto.com, Tom Horyn

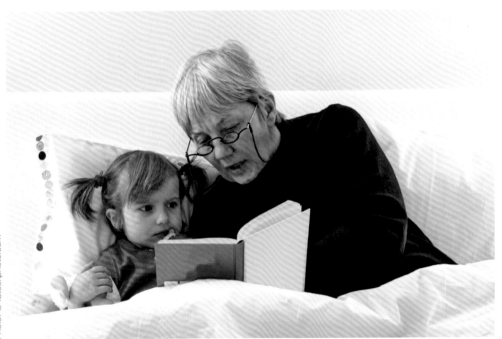

Most developed nations view contraception as sensible if not essential. Family planning is big business and we are getting good at it, with families averaging 2.5 children keeping the population more or less constant. Older people will outnumber children by four times over the next twenty years. Obviously sex and procreation are separate things to most people, especially men. Just as well, it would be standing room only for humans if late night television is anything to go by.

Pressure to have kids can come from many directions, not least the rest of the family. There is still the 'have them soon before it's too late' mentality. Even worse if the woman was older than her partner. Part of the rationale comes from the increasing danger of genetic malformations for older women and for men. (Paradoxically, more malformed children are born to much younger women simply because there is less perceived need for screening, and proportionately a lot more pregnancies.) While lambasting women for having children after menopause using modern techniques, society sees older male fathers as a positive asset. The number of kids born to women in their late 30s to 40 years is increasing by 18,000 per year. Women are voting with their wombs.

A few side-effects

Not many of us realise just how much we are going to change once there is someone else in the picture. Cash becomes more of a worry. The days of spending the pay packet within the first two days are gone forever, yet most men rate their loss of 'freedom', increased responsibility and changed sex lives more significantly than the drain on the bank account. Financial advisors reckon having children is the most expensive personal investment we will ever encounter before even buying a house. Ask any guy with a phone and teenage daughters.

Risk-taking decreases, especially when driving, and the insurance companies are quick to pick this up. During WWII unmarried young men flew the relatively cheap fighters and were encouraged to take risks while married older men, preferably with

Modern technology allows for older parents

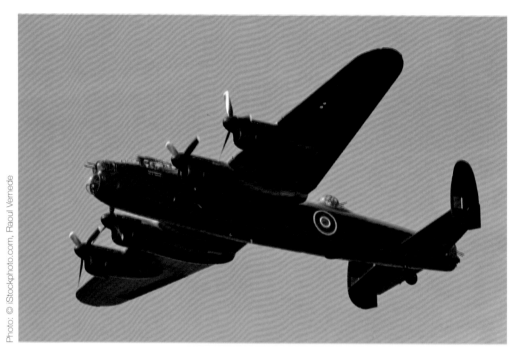

Photo: © iStockphoto.com, Raoul Vernede

children, flew the expensive bombers with their highly-trained crews. You could thus guarantee that they would do everything in their power to avoid any risk that they might not return. Pretty sneaky stuff. Even jobs in industry and the public services often reflect this shift in behaviour and most men will recognise it. When babies come along absenteeism from work declines, job migration falls, and sick leave drops.

Family men were trusted to fly the more expensive aeroplanes during the war

Babies

Whether or not your partner's pregnancy was planned, or accidental, longed for, or a nice (ish) surprise, most couples in happy relationships will find themselves becoming closer in the nine months before a baby is born. You may feel an urge to protect and look after your partner and to help her prepare the home for the new arrival. You may feel excitement at becoming a 'proper family', as well as full of anticipation about the sort of father you'll be. You'll probably be idealising yourself, your partner, and the baby. This is to be expected – you can hardly imagine the reality of having a baby before it's even arrived.

Immediately, after the birth, you may find yourself overwhelmed by the realisation that this baby is for life – from now on, you will always be a parent. This starts to hit home as you and your partner absorb the practical changes having a baby entails. Less money, interrupted sleep, no more spontaneous nights out, and a partner whose focus is very much elsewhere – it can all take their toll, especially when there is suddenly so much less time for you as a couple. All this physical change, combined with the emotional impact of the baby itself, can lead to emotional ups and downs for the two of you.

Of course, you may well feel more bonded than ever before, with a renewed determination that your relationship will last forever. Or you may be unnerved by feelings of responsibility, and these may be increased if your partner has stopped working, and seems more dependent on you that ever before. At the same time, she is probably not paying nearly as much attention to you as she used to. Although you know this is to be expected, it can leave you needing reassurance and affection, without knowing how to ask for it.

Some mothers can be possessive of their babies, and unwilling to let the father be fully involved in caring for him. Perhaps your partner even puts you down, and says you do things in the wrong way, like changing nappies. This can leave you feeling resentful, and unwanted – your relationship will certainly suffer if she does not recognise your new role as a parent. If she encourages your full participation, you will become painfully aware that your time is no longer your own. Hobbies, socialising, or simply lazing around, will now require planning, and might end up being interrupted anyway.

Another thing that will change – at least for a while – is your sex life. Very few women can, or want to, have sex in the first few weeks or months after giving birth. Even after this, she may feel uncomfortable about the changes in her body. You might find it hard to adjust to her new role as a both mother and partner, and this could change sex for you. It is vital that you concentrate on being intimate, even of you are not having sex, so that you maintain your emotional and physical bond. If you do this, your loving sexual relationship should return.

Regarding the other changes, remember to concentrate on that most important part of your software: communication. Talk about these possible changes before your partner becomes pregnant, and during the pregnancy too. Talk about what has actually happened after the baby is born – it might be a good start to compare expectations and reality together. It is important to share negative feelings as well as positive ones, and it is likely that your partner will surprise you with some negative emotions of her own. By talking them through together, you will lose the sense of pressure to be a 'perfect father', and become closer.

A final point is that you need to take time away from work to get to know your baby – maybe even without your partner there. She will probably be glad of the break. Taking some paternity leave will enable you to kick-start the bonding process with your child, by giving you the chance to take care of all his needs when he is most dependent. After that, use weekends and holidays to spend proper time with the baby. You need to bond with your baby just as much as his mother does.

If your partner is doing the night feed, enjoy the luxury of a double bed on your own, but attempt to show interest and willing by pulling back the duvet in an inviting yet-no-strings-attached manner when your she returns to the marital bed, and proceed to make weary de-milked mother feel warm and loved. You can train yourself to do this (once perfected, without actually waking up) and it never fails to please. Otherwise, be sure to ask and show compassion and gratitude to the earth-mother type whose gene pool has been mixed with your own.

Communication is important

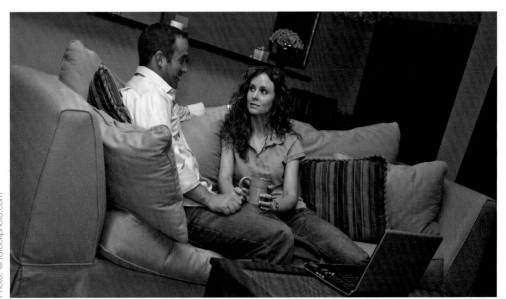

PART 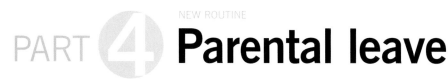 **Parental leave**

For mothers

Maternity leave entitlement has increased recently, and the mother doesn't need to have worked with her employer for a particular length of time to benefit.

- The mother can take 52 weeks maternity leave while remaining an employee, and retain the right to return to work. The employer must be notified by week 25 of the pregnancy that maternity leave will be taken.
- To get Statutory Maternity Pay (SMP) it is necessary to work for one employer continuously for at least 26 weeks, and this period must have been completed by week 25 of the pregnancy. It is also necessary to earn, before tax, an average of £87 a week.
- The first 6 weeks of SMP are paid at 90% of regular pay, the next 33 weeks are paid at £112.75 a week (unless the 90% rate is lower, in which case 90% is paid for the 39 weeks). This pay is subject to tax and national insurance contributions.
- The employer isn't legally required to provide pay for the final 13 week leave entitlement.
- The same pay and leave applies for stillbirths.
- The same pay and leave applies for the 'primary adopter' when a child is being adopted. This is Statutory Adoption Pay (SAP).
- Maternity Allowance (MA) may be payable for freelance or self-employed people; it is paid at similar levels to SMP but depends on earnings for the previous 15 months.
- Many employers are offering enhancements to the statutory maternity leave and pay.

For fathers

New fathers seem to get a bit of a raw deal, legally, compared to mothers.

- To get Statutory Paternity Pay (SPP) it is necessary to work for one employer continuously for at least 26 weeks, and this period must have been completed by week 25 of the pregnancy.
- Leave entitlement is 2 weeks regardless of length of time with the employer. The employer can require this is taken in one block, or two separate weeks.
- During the 2 weeks leave SPP is £112.75 a week, or 90% of average weekly earnings if this is less. These payments are subject to tax and national insurance contributions.
- The same pay and leave applies for stillbirths.
- The same pay and leave applies for adoption, and the leave is normally taken within the first 56 days of adoption.
- Some employers are offering enhancements to the statutory paternity pay although (so far) not the leave.

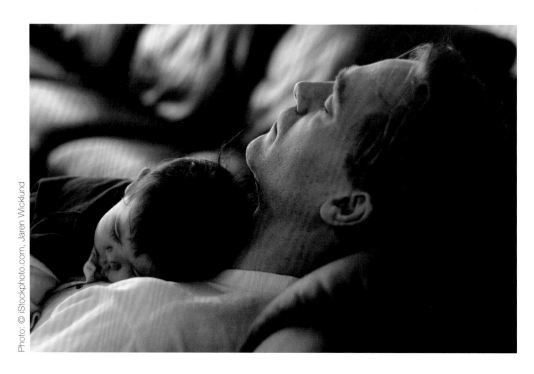

Photo: © iStockphoto.com, Jaren Wicklund

PART 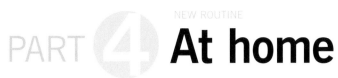 **At home**

Introduction

Your baby will have been seen, handled, admired and checked by everyone in the ward, doctors, midwives, relatives and possibly clergy. Now, at home you have him or her to yourselves. It is a time of great peace, but possibly short-lived. Soon you will have the relatives, well-wishers, neighbours and all the back-up services of modern medicine beating a path to your door. Be warned, well-wishing phone callers will want to know about how your partner is, how well is the baby and did the baby cry when introduced to the world, before they ask about your crushed fingers, your part of the birth support team. Fathers, on the Richter scale of childbirth, feature low in the table of concern.

Kids in the house

Having another competitor entering the pool is not always good news. Simply telling a child that from now on there will be another brother or sister in the house is the equivalent of informing a politician that a new candidate, younger and more attractive, has set up office in their backyard. Don't expect thanks. It is an unfortunate analogy, but there is the politician's equivalent of the 'sweetener' when it comes to helping children accept the idea of a new addition to the family. To simply expect them to welcome diluted attention from the most important

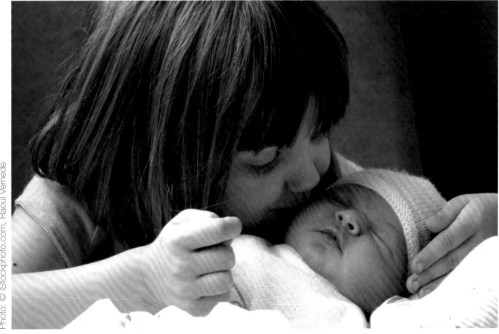

Photo: © iStockphoto.com, Raoul Vernede

people in their lives is wishful thinking. The average child can hate a newcomer to the family with a ferocity matched only by companies competing for the same contract. By showing attention to the older child, reassuring them that they are still loved and wanted just as much as ever, that their mummy and daddy brought along this new baby for them to play with is infinitely better than ignoring their feeling of insecurity. If a small present in celebration of the event happens to be one that the older child can play with along with the new addition, so what? You, your partner, and anyone within range will be invited to join in the celebration with food, drink and happiness, why not the one who perceives they have most to lose?

Baby blues

It was once dismissed as myth, but baby blues can also hit the dad as well as the mum. There is plenty of help available to you and your partner. Your GP, community midwife, social worker and health visitor will all be sources of good advice and help. Naturally the new mum will feel exhausted and emotionally drained. For some this feeling not only fails to lift but can actually become worse and is called postnatal depression. Telling your partner to 'snap out of it' or to 'pull yourself together' is not only bound to make things worse but also increases strain on your relationship. Other children in the house will be quick to notice these changes and may interpret them as not wanting the new baby. In severe cases, which are thankfully rare, it may need the attention of the family doctor. Postnatal depression is not the same as the common, some would call normal, phenomenon of the two-day baby blues. Weeping for no apparent reason is common about two or three days after the baby is born. It rarely lasts more than a day or so but it helps to understand that nothing serious, other than emotional and hormonal changes, are involved.

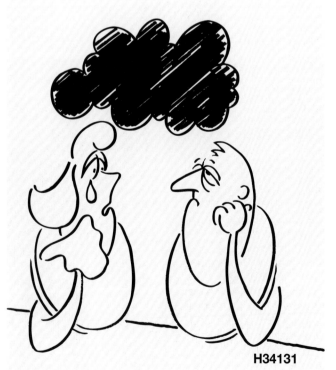

H34131

Getting back home

Many people are superstitious about leaving the hospital without their child. Similarly, relatives and friends are always unsure what they should do if the baby has some malformation or may even have died. Celebration, with empathy for the mother's grieving, is better than total silence when there is some problem with the baby. Talking about a 'club' foot or a Down's syndrome is better than simply trying to ignore it. All kinds of emotion will surface for the father to cope with, from his partner, himself and relatives. Unjustified feelings of guilt and shame are common. Many mothers feel as though it has been their fault and they will look for possible reasons. A fall, a recent stressful event, or alcohol taken during pregnancy will all be whips with which to beat herself. Fathers will often not feel free of this self-guilt, but talking and reassuring is constructive, while taking part in the self reproach is not. Rejection of you as a father is paradoxically not uncommon. It needs to be talked through and there is expert help available from your maternity unit, but also look at the addresses at the end of the book.

Will things ever be the same again?

For many fathers, the homecoming is a conflict of emotions. Far from being the fulfilment and permanent party atmosphere, strain on the relationship can be a major factor. Lack of sleep, uncertainty over the future and confusion over the division of affection all contribute to a feeling of 'unreality'. Many men will take off a few days from work to help their partner settle back home, despite the fact that there is a lamentable lack of parental leave for such occasions (see *Parental leave* on page 78). Yet for some, if they are completely honest, it will be a relief to get back to work. Even so, returning to work when tired and trying to help at home with feeding and looking after the baby, will also place a strain on your relationship. All those books and ante-natal courses with their parent craft do not seem to apply to you and your baby. Only *your* baby cries for 23 hours per day, needs feeding seven times in the night and nobody else's partner treats you like a Martian. In truth, give or take the extraterrestrial reference, this is par for the course, but it gets better.

Returning to work is only the beginning. Work has not ceased when you leave your place of employment. Suddenly it is impossible to go out with friends, cinema and the theatre are fond memories. Even intimate moments with your partner can be interrupted or take place in bed next to a baby-gro which appears to contain a small octopus. Mixed feelings prevail. Self-fulfilment fights for supremacy with sadness over the loss of freedom. Like most things of any importance in a relationship, talking to your partner about your needs, the possible use of a baby-sitter, going out individually or simply staying at home and making it even more attractive, is the best way of approaching this common dilemma.

Better sex

There is no biological reason why you cannot resume intercourse as soon as both of you wish to do so. Common-sense dictates that the presence of stitches, if an episiotomy has been repaired, will not make the experience something to look forward to, particularly by your partner. For some men there is a period of being 'turned off' by the whole experience. This is seldom a major problem and as things return to as near normal as they will ever be, given that there is someone else in the equation from now on, sexual relationships invariably improve. The same thing is obviously true for your partner, and disregarding her feelings will only serve to add more strain on the relationship. As with sex during pregnancy, there can be ways of making sex more enjoyable, or even possible, after the birth of the baby. Different positions, a cushion under her hips or lying side-by-side may help. Lubricating gels can overcome the dryness of the vagina which may follow from the change in hormones and can be more common with breastfeeding. Libido you both enjoyed before the baby may not be the same afterwards but like swings and roundabouts, there are gains and losses. In the main, the losses are temporary while the gains are permanent.

Post birth contraception

It is probably fair to say that most men, and women, are not considering another child immediately after the birth. After what they have just been through, it is probably the last thing your partner is considering.

There are some myths surrounding conception after childbirth:

It is impossible to conceive until after the first period

Untrue, an egg can be released from the ovary before the first period, as many couples with closely-spaced children will testify.

It is impossible to conceive while breastfeeding

In some circumstances breastfeeding is 98% effective as a contraceptive – the baby must be less than six months old, the women should not have had a period yet and the baby must *only* be having breast milk regularly day and night. Relatively soon after the birth one of these factors usually changes so contraception is needed even if breastfeeding continues.

Your partner cannot take the pill until she stops breastfeeding

Not true, although any drug or hormone can affect her milk production while breastfeeding, so it's best to talk with your doctor.

Hormones in the pill will affect the baby, particularly if it is a boy, when breastfeeding

There is little evidence that these hormones harm either sex of baby in the tiny quantities that are present in breast milk. Even so some women may prefer to avoid any medicines or drugs during breastfeeding and use an alternative form of contraception.

What to feel

For a number of fathers there is a flat emotional response to the baby after it arrives home. They can feel guilty that they are not continuously enraptured by their baby. For many fathers, however, they consider the real development in the relationship with their baby when the child begins to respond or to smile in recognition. It appears that men crave recognition of their presence when that of the mother is only too obvious.

For some fathers, there is a link between a positive attitude towards the new baby and stable partnerships. Positive memories of activities with their own fathers are also important. While this may seem obvious, if true it means that fathers who did not have such a good relationship with their own fathers may at first experience some difficulty in forming their own immediate relationships with the new baby. Even for these fathers, the recognition of their presence by their baby usually initiates a cascade of emotions which overcomes much of the initial inhibition.

Enjoy your baby while they are young because as soon as they become mobile your life will become increasingly hard.

Financial concerns

Few men have the luxury in the present economic climate of being 100% sure of a steadily increasing income. Yet the perception of having children is the need for more money. Unfortunately, this is never more true than for the first child. In fact there is a greater demand on the home for money and concerns over finance can very easily cloud the enjoyment of a new child, and can be expressed in different ways such as apparent indifference, lack of patience and even excessive drinking which doesn't seem to stop after the initial celebrations of the birth of the baby.

Breasts aren't what they used to be

Where men have expressed concern or given reasons against breastfeeding they admit to:

- Honest jealousy.
- Less involvement with the baby if the father cannot give bottles.
- A desire to see the woman return to normal weight and energy.
- A revulsion at leaking and heavy breasts.

There are no easy answers, and each of these reasons has its own built-in agenda of previous experience. While men harbour these concerns they often fail to discuss them with someone else, not least their own partner. Jealousy for attention is common and can be addressed by actually talking to each other. Not 'getting a look in' with regard to feeding the new baby is similarly a common emotion, and can be expressed in ways apparently unconnected to the cause. Bad temper and lack of patience during feeding times are common manifestations of irritation. This can be overcome to some extent by allowing more 'cuddle time' but also by bottle feeding with expressed milk. This can have enormous benefits when the time comes for some intimate time alone and the baby can be looked after for a short time by a relative. Revulsion over the appearance and function of your partner's breasts is equally common and may even be of biological value in protecting the food source of the baby. This revulsion can even extend to the vagina which, to some men, may 'never seem the same again'.

Tactful discussion with your partner is better than innuendo which leaves both of you wondering about your mutual attraction. Like the pain of childbirth itself, these changes have a finite duration. Such is the power of human sexual attraction, these feeling rarely become permanent obstacles to sexual relationships.

Men too!

Female baby blues and postnatal depression are very real phenomena and have rightly received attention from both the medical profession and the media. But whereas society will sympathise with a woman suffering from, say, postnatal depression (PND), it is much more difficult for a man to admit to this problem. Few men would consult their GP and even fewer would ask for time off work and, while we may be getting better

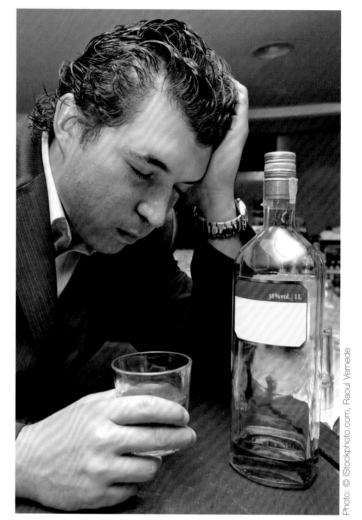

Photo: © iStockphoto.com, Raoul Vernede

at it, rather than analyse and discuss the problem, many men will demonstrate sometimes subtle, sometimes dramatic changes in their normal routine. Drinking can be a serious attempt at consolation which seldom if ever gives even temporary relief. Men need to understand that like women they can suffer from a similar form of depression, that they are not alone with their ambivalence and that all around them, in the workplace, in the neighbourhood, there are other men with similar emotional needs.

Emotional 'burnout' and its prevention

Burnout is probably a good term to describe what happens when a person gets an overload of responsibility, worry and fear for the safety of other people. It can also happen to men who have become fathers. A major factor is not just the severity of the pressure but its perceived 'open-endedness'. When such unremitting pressure is felt to be unending, people can rapidly become depressed. With the emotional trauma of childbirth, the lack of sleep, financial implications along with the effect it can be having upon relationships with their partner, it is perhaps not surprising that many men can be affected.

Even the most dedicated worker, teacher, artist, whatever, will admit the need for some time away from it, and parenthood is no exception. During the first two or three months it may be very difficult to find enough time between feeds to go out for an entire evening. It is necessary to organise some form of social support, for fathers as well as mothers. Feeling that they are the only people who feel this way is common, yet with the arrival of the new baby a whole population of men and women appear who have the same emotional strains and can support each other.

With some foresight, it is possible to work out a programme for time-sharing and there is an increasing number of fathers who are so deeply convinced that their role is equal to that of mothers that they take an extended leave from work. In most parts of Europe there is legal provision to do just this. Sometimes this is for practical reasons, because the mother's salary is higher, or because the father is in an easier position to take a break from his work.

As this arrangement becomes more acceptable, fathers are expressing specific needs in coping with being at home. Like women, men can also be lonely at home and need emotional and practical support. All the dilemma of isolation at home, lack of sufficient stimulus and the feeling of aimlessness can be a common complaint of men who may have anticipated few such problems. Obviously there is little difference here between men and women.

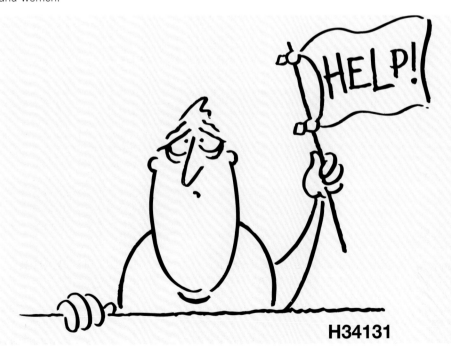

H34131

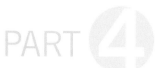

Dads have feelings too!

Looking after ourselves as fathers

Being a father can often be great fun and really rewarding – although it can also be stressful and demanding. Kids can take up so much of our time and energy that we don't pay much attention to what we're really feeling.

This Section looks at the kinds of things we go through as dads, and discusses the benefits which talking and thinking about the ups and downs of being a dad can have on our own lives and on the lives of our kids.

The feelings we have as a dad

Having a range of different feelings is natural. They come and go and vary in strength depending on the situation. As parents it's really important that we're aware of what we're feeling and can recognise when our feelings are getting on top of us. Children are very aware of how their parents feel, and this can affect them and their behaviour.

How we feel about being a dad depends on lots of things:

- Our personality and temperament.
- Whether we have the support of a partner, family and friends.
- How many children we have, and what ages and stages they're at.
- How physically and mentally healthy they are.
- Whether we're combining child care with paid work.
- Whether we have enough money to bring up our family or are worried about money.
- Whether we live in comfortable housing or are struggling with poor accommodation.
- Whether we're coping with stressful events in our lives such as a separation, a bereavement or unemployment.
- The experiences we had in our own childhood, and whether or not we have been able to come to terms with any problems that we faced when we were young.

Being a father can often be great fun and really rewarding – although it can also be stressful and demanding. Kids can take up so much of our time and energy

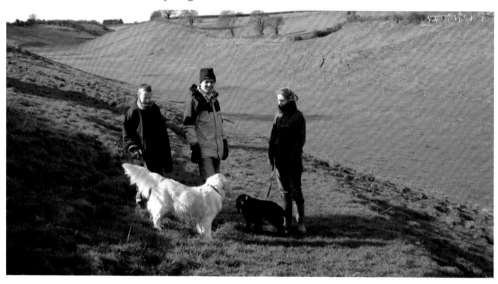

An important part of being a dad is the ability to be sensitive and responsive to our kids' emotions. Children experience and express strong emotions and that can sometimes be quite challenging for us as adults. We may have been brought up to deny the full range of our feelings, and can be surprised at how powerfully they can come back when we're bringing up our own children. As well as loving and caring for our children, there may also be times when we struggle with difficult feelings such as:

● Anger.
● Resentment.
● Exhaustion.
● Envy.
● Boredom.
● Guilt.
● Sadness.
● Disappointment.
● Despair.

Although it can be painful to acknowledge our more negative feelings, it is helpful to try and make sense of how we react, so that we can take steps to look after ourselves and enjoy the good aspects of being a parent.

When we become parents some of the things we say or do might remind us of the way our own parents treated us when we were children. Although some of these reactions may be helpful, we may also find ourselves repeating more destructive behaviour. For example, if our own parents were unable to control their anger, we might lose our temper with our children more often than we would like. Or, we may make a real effort to parent in a more positive way but then we may feel a bit jealous or resentful because our children are having a much easier childhood than we did.

It's also important to remember that there's no such thing as a perfect mum or dad, we all have good and bad days and we all make mistakes.

Our feelings at different stages of being a dad

Our experiences and needs as parents will change over time depending on the age and developmental stage of our children.

Pregnancy

This can be a time of change, great stress, or even crisis, for expectant fathers. Quite a large percentage of fathers get depressed or anxious during their partner's pregnancy; these are quite natural reactions – perhaps we might be feeling worried about how we'll cope with bringing up a child, or anxious about what effect the child will have on our relationship with our partner? It is important to listen to ourselves – there may be a lot of joy around the idea of a new child, but it may also bring sadness (perhaps the new child will mean the end, in some sense, of our own 'childhood', for example). It's important to realize that it's ok to feel these things.

Getting involved in caring for our child can help us feel more confident about what we can offer

After the birth

Dads need time, support and encouragement to develop bonds with the child. We can often feel left out of childcare because, just as with first-time mothers, we don't have the skills.

Maybe our partner, or someone else in the family has said things like this to us? If we feel unsure of our new role, and unsupported by those around us, we may react by trying to

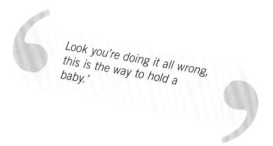

'I feel a bit worried when you throw her up in the air that way. Babies have delicate necks and she might get hurt.'

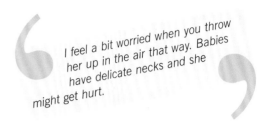

'Look you're doing it all wrong, this is the way to hold a baby.'

pretend that nothing's happening, and trying to get things back to how they were before the birth. Or perhaps we'll find ourselves spending more time with our friends, and that this leads to

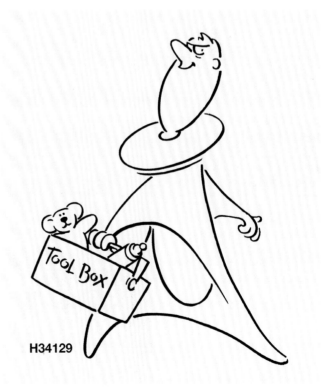

H34129

arguments with our partner. It's important to recognize that whilst it's healthy to have a bit of space now and then from the baby, becoming distant, or withdrawing physically and emotionally isn't going to help us, our baby or our partner in the long run. Getting more involved in caring for our child can help us feel more confident about what we can offer.

Grandparents can often be a great source of help when we're trying to bring up children. But maybe we feel they're focusing so much on the baby that they don't really see us, our partner and the baby as a new family? Although this can be painful, it's very common for there to be tensions amongst families at such times. The arrival of a baby means that everyone has to adjust their place and position in the family (our own parents will become grandparents, with all the mixed feelings that may bring, for example), and this can be quite painful sometimes.

Being the father of a young child

As the father of a young child, you may have to deal with some difficult, painful feelings around how close the bond is between your child and the mother of the child – when the child is very young, you may feel quite left out, and begin to wonder when you'll be able to bond with your child in the way that your partner has. And in spite of these feelings, your partner will probably be expecting a lot of support from you. It's at times like these that you may feel sad that you have to go to work every day and can't see your daughter or son during the day; there's always a danger though that feelings like these are too painful to experience, and so we end up getting angry or pretending we're not interested.

It's also very often the case that a mum and dad of a child will have different views at times about how to be a parent. This can lead to rows and unhappiness if you find that you are often at odds with your partner. However, it's worth remembering that no one way of parenting is always 'right', and that your opinions about how best to do things are as important as anyone else's.

A young child will look to their parents as role models. A dad who is capable of managing his emotions – being able to deal with your own anger, for example, by keeping things together, and not yelling or shouting; or being able to admit to feelings of disappointment or frustration, rather than bottling them up, and denying them – will provide your son or daughter with a really helpful example of how to be a mature person who can understand and deal with the range of feelings that come about during the course of everyday life.

Being the father of a teenager

Being the father of a teenager can be tough going at times. Although it can be really great to see your child start to express their own opinions and tastes, and begin to have an independent life, it can also be difficult to know how to relate to them. Teenagers grow up quickly, and it can be difficult to know how to allow them greater freedom while still setting the usual boundaries to make sure that they stay safe. Some days you may not even see your teenage son or daughter for more than a few minutes, especially if they're often in their room with their friends, on the computer or listening to music, or if they spend a lot of time elsewhere. Good communication and negotiation skills are needed at this time! Much depends on how your teenager is coping with the stresses of being that age. It's important to stay in touch with them even though they may be very rejecting at times, which can be quite painful for us as parents. Try to reflect on how your son or daughter might view you – are you being too strict or too lenient? Are you letting them become individuals, or do you end up fighting the same battles about staying out too long, not doing homework, etc?

Increasingly interested in, and loyal to young people his or her own age, your teenage son or daughter will probably struggle to admit to just how much they want and need your love and approval – it's an age where these kinds of feelings don't sit very easily with the desire for independence and freedom. It takes a lot of self-belief to be able to carry on believing just how important you are for your teenager – but in spite of all the evidence they provide to the contrary, your teenage children still need you!

Being a step-father

If you are a step-father to a child or a number of children, the information and advice in this Section is just as relevant to you as to biological fathers. However, being a step-father can bring particular stresses. For example, it can be very painful if you feel that your partner's children are rejecting you, particularly when you are going out of your way to get along with them. Your step-children have probably been through some sad and distressing times and may be missing their biological father. Perhaps they feel they are being disloyal to their father if they are friendly with you. It's bound to be a very complex situation which needs a lot of time and patience to settle down, and one which may well demand a lot from you in terms of your ability to remain positive, even in the face of anger and resentment. You may also need to reassure any children you may have from a previous relationship that you still love them and will always be their father. You may feel disappointed that you don't get to spend as much time alone with your partner as you would like and find yourself resenting your step-children. It's not uncommon to have these kind of feelings and it may be a good idea to talk to your partner about how you're feeling and how difficult the situation can be.

Continuing to be a father after a divorce or separation

If your children are living with their mother after a divorce or separation, having to deal with the restrictions placed on you about where and how often you can see them can be distressing and even feel humiliating. You may be very angry about how little time you are allowed with them, or resent the fact that you can't be spontaneous and turn up and see them when you like. No-one can pretend that handling these kind of situations and emotions is anything but difficult. But looking after yourself includes trying not to let your feelings overwhelm you and spoil the most important thing – your relationship with your kids.

How to recognise when we are in trouble

It's important to recognise the difference between feelings which are very natural responses to the stresses and struggles of bringing up children and feelings which are beginning to interfere with our ability to cope.

Everyone has bad days and some of the symptoms of mental health difficulties may not immediately seem obvious. Take a look at the list below – do any of these sound familiar?

- Having difficulty getting to sleep, or waking up early and not being able to get back to sleep again.
- Feeling really tired even when you haven't really done much.
- Getting aches and pains for no obvious reason or feeling run down.
- Not having much appetite.
- Not feeling like going out.
- Not being interested in the things you were interested in before.
- Feeling anxious and tetchy for no real reason, or 'flying off the handle' a lot.
- Getting lots of headaches or migraines.

If they do, then you should probably consider taking some of the steps in the next paragraphs.

How can I look after my mental health?

Sometimes our problems can feel too much or too difficult to manage by ourselves. Talking to a friend or a family member about what's getting to us is a useful way to let off steam, and often helps to reduce stress.

But sometimes it may not be easy to talk to friends or family; at these times it can be helpful to talk to someone who is outside of our daily lives. Your GP should be able to put you in touch with a professional such as-a counsellor or psychotherapist – who can offer the chance to go over current or past difficulties, problems and emotions, and help you to move forward. If you are feeling very depressed, your GP may offer you anti-depressants which may be helpful in the short-term if you feel so low that you are unable to cope. However, it is important to try to understand why you are feeling depressed in the hope that you can makes some changes to your situation. It is always worth asking if you can be referred to a professional.

Going to see a counsellor or a psychotherapist doesn't mean you're mad – in fact, it shows that you're interested in helping yourself, and that you want to make sense of how you feel. It's a very positive step to take. If you just carry on feeling upset or stressed, and things aren't getting any better, or they're getting worse, you're going to be less use to your partner and to your children. They need you to be available for them, and taking steps to make yourself feel better is a really sensible thing to do.

That's not to say though that talking about what's upsetting us is easy. It can feel like we're losing control, letting everything spill out. Or it can feel difficult as we're worried about what they'll think of us. But remember, unless we take care of our own needs, we can't truly be in the right frame of mind either to give love or to receive it.

Looking after your physical health can help your mental health

Looking after our physical health can help our mental health – the two things are much more connected than most people realize. For example, the food that we eat has a direct effect on our mood. So, it's worth trying to have a well balanced diet which includes plenty of fresh fruit and vegetables. Plus, exercising, and making sure we get enough sleep (kids permitting!), helps us to release tension and stay physically well. Also, keeping our feelings bottled up inside can be very stressful, and can also lead to physical symptoms such as headaches and digestive problems – so it's best to make sure we can talk to someone about how we feel (see above). Lastly, it's important to give ourselves a break from the children. This will help us be better dads, and we shouldn't feel guilty about having a bit of time and space to ourselves now and then.

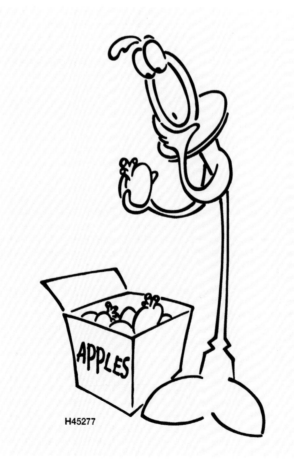

H45277

Try to have a well balanced diet which includes plenty of fresh fruit and vegetables

Cot death

Also known as Sudden Infant Death Syndrome (SIDS) the sudden death of infants while in their cots is still a mystery but there are some recognised ways of preventing these tragedies.

As with any bereavement, disbelief and denial are just as strong after a cot death, but the feeling of guilt is perhaps even more prevalent. All the more sad because in truth we do not know what causes a cot death, but this will not prevent bereaved parents from mercilessly whipping themselves as if they could somehow have prevented it from happening. Media attention on smoking, alcohol or the temperature of the room only serve to reinforce the feeling of misplaced guilt. Anger is common, directed at almost anyone, but sadly it can be levelled at the person who needs the complete opposite, your partner.

Symptoms

Generally the baby, usually between 3 and 18 months old, is found dead after being laid down to sleep with no signs of distress.

Causes

The cause of sudden death of infants is still a mystery, but a lot of work has been done to try and prevent future tragedies. No clearly identifiable cause is known although there are recognised risk factors, so it is possible to reduce the risk of it happening.

Diagnosis

Deciding on the cause of death can be very traumatic for parents. In truth we do not know why it happens and can only suggest ways of helping preventing it happening again. It is not an indictment of the parents.

Coming to terms with a cot death takes a long time and few people ever really 'get over it' but simply learn how to deal with the feeling of loss. No better time to be gentle with your partner and yourself. Some bereaved fathers find counselling helpful while others prefer to handle it on their own. Without doubt the best way of coming to terms with it all is to talk about it to someone who is not judgmental and is quite prepared to listen to the same unanswerable questions over and over again. For men, these gifted people can unfortunately be hard to find and the age old macho 'pull yourself together' technique is inevitably applied.

Prevention

- Put your baby on their back to sleep, not on their stomach ('Back To Bed')
- Do not smoke in the house, and encourage others not to do so.
- Babies are more likely to overheat than to get too cold and will not always make a noise. Avoid overheating them by using minimal covers and clothes. If they are hot, cool them with ventilation, by taking off their covers and by reducing the temperature of the room. Don't keep tucking them in if they throw the covers off - this may be a sign that they are too hot.
- Be alert to the danger of overheating in cars, shops etc.
- If possible, move the cot into your bedroom, but avoid sleeping with the baby in your bed.

Treatment

Extra precautions with your new baby could include:
- Have your baby weighed and measured regularly.
- Convince your partner and visitors about the danger of smoking in the house.

Don't smoke in the house. (Even better, don't smoke at all!)

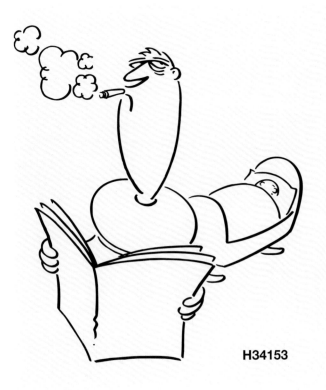

H34153

PART 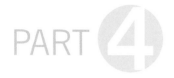 # Feeding

Breastfeeding

Breastfeeding gives both the mother and the baby many more advantages than formula milk. It is natural, free and convenient and is designed specifically for the needs of your baby.

Did you know that?
Babies who are breastfed have:
- Less risk of sickness and diarrhoea.
- Fewer ear infections.
- Fewer chest infections.
- Less risk of allergies such as asthma, eczema.
- Less likely to become obese in childhood.
- Less likely to develop diabetes.

Breastfeeding also gives the mother many health benefits too:
- Women who breastfeed are at less risk of developing breast and ovarian cancer and have better protection against developing osteoporosis.

Breast milk is convenient and free:
- No need to sterilise, make up and warm bottles.
- No need to buy formula milk.
- Kinder to the environment.

How does breastfeeding work?
- Milk is produced by cells in the mother's breast and then ejected in response to hormones that are produced by the mother as the baby suckles at her breast.
- The more the baby feeds the more milk is produced.
- The baby needs to be attached and positioned well at the breast in order to feed effectively.

Breast fed babies will get the squits if you eat curry, and wind if you drink orange juice.

The baby needs to be properly attached to the breast

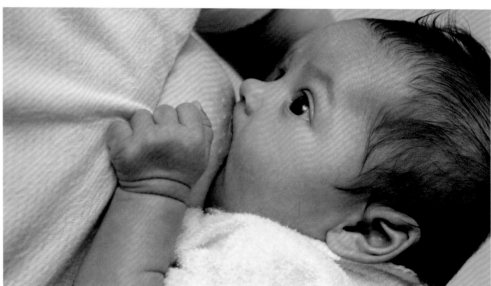

Photo: © iStockphoto.com, Gloria-Leigh Logan

- Nipple soreness or pain during feeding is usually a sign that the baby is not attached correctly at the breast.
- If the mother is comfortable and relaxed, she and the baby are more likely to enjoy feeding.
- Breastfed babies usually feed frequently (maybe every 2 to 3 hours) in the early weeks and many babies feed even more frequently in the evenings.
- Nighttime feeds are important for the production of enough milk for the following day.
- Babies are usually more settled and less windy if they finish one breast first and then finish off the feed with the second breast.
- Breast milk provides the baby with all the nutrition it requires for the first 6 months of life.
- A breast fed baby does not require any extra drinks of water even in hot weather.

Do fathers really make a difference?
Yes: A woman is more likely to choose to breastfeed if she is sure her partner is positive about it.

How can fathers help with breastfeeding?
- Help build your partner's confidence by reassuring and praising her.
- Even though you can't breastfeed, be involved in the care of your baby in other ways, eg, bathing, changing nappy, winding, taking for walks, playing and talking.
- Help your partner with the household chores and caring for older children.
- Encourage your partner to eat and drink regularly so she will feel more able to cope.
- Talk and listen to each other about how you feel about having a new baby.
- If your partner is experiencing difficulties, encourage her to get professional help.

Screaming babies almost always have wind and the best cure is to put a linen cloth on your left shoulder, put the baby on your shoulder so they can see around (chin on your shoulder) and pat the baby's back 3 times followed by a circular comforting motion. Repeat until baby is comfortable, and take your time, they always save some. You must pat firmly but not hard. Later in life the child will find this motion very comforting when they get upset. For left-handed people use your right shoulder. Baby will learn the difference between mum and dad.

Never try to wind baby lying down, if you can't stand up to do this put the linen over your left-hand (for right-handed people), use the bridge of your thumb and forefinger to support the baby's chin then pat and rub in the same way. Baby can sit on your lap. Beware though if the baby slumps forward it will compress the stomach and they will almost certainly puke.

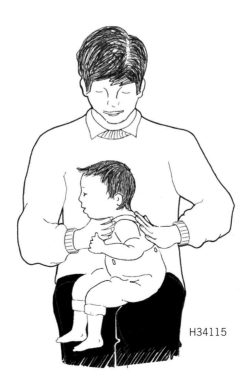

Winding: simply rubbing the baby's back after feeds is enough to help them settle

H34115

Common concerns of fathers

I am worried that I won't feel as involved with the baby.
Fathers can sometimes feel jealous of the closeness that
the mother and baby share during feeding. This closeness
is really important for the emotional development of your
baby. However you will be able to be involved in many other
important roles.

Eventually, after several weeks, your partner may be able
to express some breast milk and you may be able to feed it to
the baby. It is important that your baby is not introduced to a
teat until breastfeeding is going successfully. It is important to
try not to use formula milk in replacement for a breast feed, as
this will affect the amount of milk your partner will produce.

**I am worried that I will feel embarrassed about my partner
breastfeeding.**
Many fathers feel like this before their baby is born but feel
very different once your baby has arrived and needs feeding.

Babies can be fed very discreetly in public; in fact most
people won't even realise a baby is being fed nearby. A lot of
shops and public buildings provide facilities for mothers to
feed their baby.

Will our sex life be affected by breastfeeding?
Having a new baby affects most couples' sex life no matter
what method of feeding they choose. Breastfeeding can cause
vaginal dryness in some women so a lubricant gel may help.

Breast stimulation can cause milk to be ejected so a towel
on hand may be useful. Feeding the baby before having sex
will help reduce this.

Although exclusive breastfeeding can have a contraceptive
effect this cannot be relied on, so contraception is essential if
you are not ready for another baby just yet.

Many women actually find that their sex drive increases
during breastfeeding!

Feel proud!
You and your partner will be able to feel great pride in the fact
that by choosing to breastfeed your baby you have given him the
best possible start in life.

Bottle feeding

When it comes to food for babies, breast is best, but for some
couples there will be no choice and for various reasons bottle
feeding is the only option. It is unfair blaming mothers when they
choose or have no choice but to bottle feed. It is more difficult
to go from bottle feed to breastfeeding than *vice versa*. There
are two selfish aspects to all this for men. Bottle feeding gives
you a chance to be part of the equation and there are few things
that you can do which will bring you closer to your baby. On the
other hand, breastfeeding frees the man to do other things and is
particularly tempting when night feeds are on the go.

There was once a school of thought, much favoured by
disciplinarians, that babies should feed and be fed when told to.
Not surprisingly this produced a lot of very noisy babies and loss
of scalp hair amongst parents. As with breastfeeding, babies are
the best judge of when they are hungry and how much food they
need. This will vary from day to day and not taking a full bottle is

There is no reason to feel
guilty about inability or
your choice not to breast
feed. Take no notice of the
staff in the hospital, or
their patronising posters.
If you can't or won't that's
your choice.

Using a typical cold water steriliser

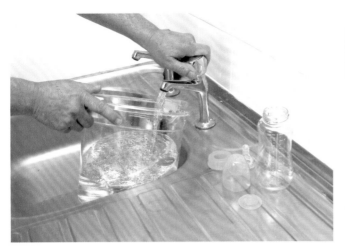

1 Fill the unit with cold water to the level mark indicated

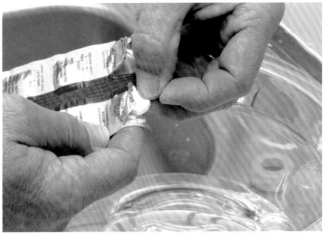

2 Add the required amount of sterilising solution or tablet

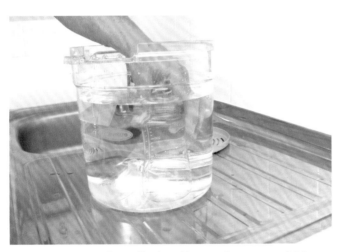

3 Insert the items to be sterilised, making sure they are completely covered and free from bubbles

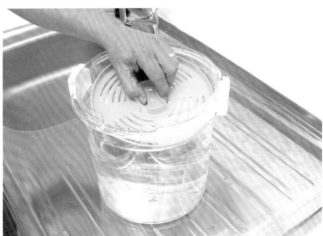

4A Cover with the sinker plate . . .

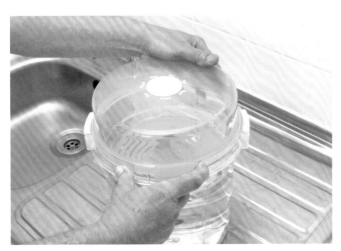

4B . . . and fit the lid

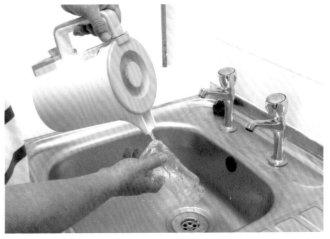

5 Rinse sterilised items before use with water which has been boiled and allowed to cool

no sign of impending disaster, often they will take more the next feed.

Advantages of breast milk
- Antibodies present give early protection from infections.
- Less constipation.
- Contains exactly the correct nutrients and fluids in exactly the right proportion.
- Easily digested with less chance of gastroenteritis.
- Less chance of allergies.
- Automatically changes in composition as the baby matures.
- Less chance of obesity, in childhood and in adult life too.
- Comes at exactly the right temperature.
- There is now evidence that breastfeeding also protects the mother from some serious medical conditions in later life.

The only disadvantages for some men is the appearance of their partner's breasts. For other men this just happens to be a real turn-on.

How to bottle feed
Choose somewhere comfy and have everything ready before starting.

Get the temperature right, drip some on the inside of your wrist. Too hot is far worse than too cool as many babies will guzzle away on cool milk. Microwave ovens are great for vegetables but not for heating babies bottles. There is a variation in temperature through the milk, and it can even be very hot without the outside of the bottle even getting warm.

What not to do
Don't keep the remaining milk for later feeds.

Crying after feeds might not be hunger, but thirst instead. Try cooled boiled water on its own but make sure the bottle is sterilised first.

Don't rush things. Taking a nap in the middle of a feed is common. The baby might take one as well.

> Sucking in air will give your baby wind, so tilt the bottle to keep the teat full of milk. A too small hole in the teat will frustrate them, and too large will cause an overflow.

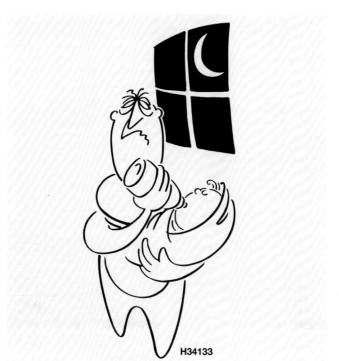

H34133

> There is nothing to be gained from Mum and Dad both attending the child or being awake during night feeds. Take it in turns to get up to the baby and be considerate to your partner. They need sleep too. A good tip is to have a sofa or comfy chair in the baby's room and comfortable lighting. Never take a screaming baby back to the bedroom unless you need your partner's help.

Preparing a bottle feed

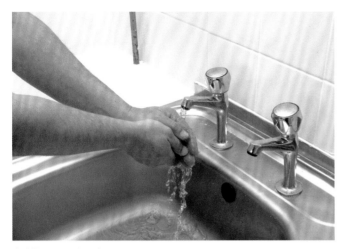

1 Wash your hands

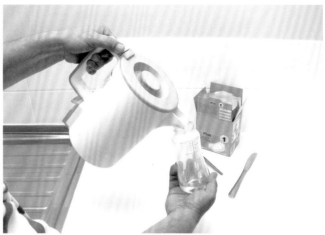

2 Boil some fresh water in a kettle or saucepan and allow to cool. Fill a previously sterilised bottle to the correct mark on the bottle according to the instructions on the packet

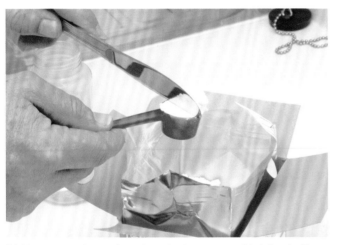

3A Measure out the powder using only the scoop provided. Level with a clean knife . . .

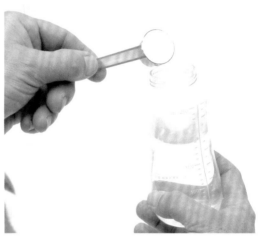

3B . . . and add to the bottle

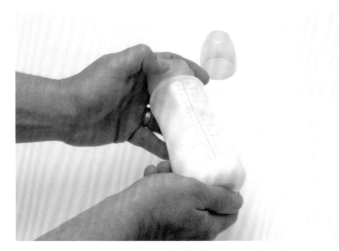

4 Replace the cap and shake well until all the powder has dissolved

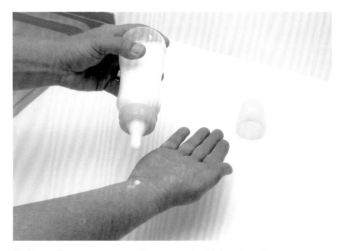

5 Test milk temperature against your wrist. Enjoy, time of night allowing

PART 4 Sterilisers

Keeping the bottles clean and free from old milk is important, but they must also be sterilised. A good scrub in hot water with washing up liquid will get rid of any food left inside, then you have a choice of sterilising methods:

- **Chemical**. These consist of a tank containing sterilising solution in which the bottles are immersed.
- **Steam**. Much quicker.
- **Microwave**. This holds the bottle in the microwave oven in such a way as to completely sterilise the inside, but this requires a special microwave sterilising chamber.

Size matters

Babies who are fully bottle-fed require at least six bottles a day so you will need a steriliser which holds at least this many bottles. Not surprisingly therefore, sterilisers come with varying capacity – from two to eight bottles. It is worth erring on the side of the larger capacity or buy the faster systems as babies can be very unforgiving when forced to wait with an empty tummy.

Cold water sterilisers

These require sterilising tablets or liquid. You will need to leave bottles, teats, etc, in the soaking solution for at least 30 minutes and they will remain sterile if kept in the soaking solution for up to 24 hours. You should discard this solution after 24 hours and make up a fresh batch. Do not use bottles directly from the steriliser. Always rinse in cooled previously-boiled water first.

Microwave sterilisers

As you would expect, these require no chemicals or rinsing and simply kill any bacteria by using steam heat not the microwaves themselves. Depending on the wattage of the microwave, it generally takes around 3-8 minutes which is much more convenient than the cold water system but metal cutlery, for instance, cannot be sterilised in a microwave.

Electric steam sterilisers

Like the microwave system, these require no chemicals or rinsing and need only water and an electrical supply as they kill bacteria using steam heat. Sterilising takes 6-15 minutes and items remain sterile for 1-24 hours depending on unit.

Microwave ovens are not always a good way of sterilising babies' bottles

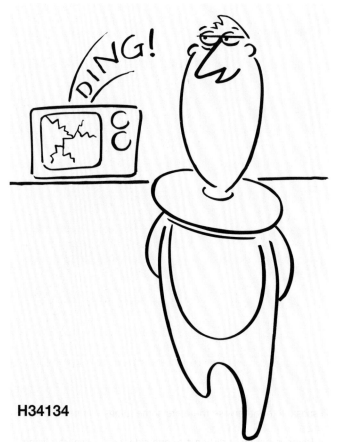

H34134

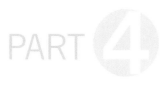

Nappies/diapers and skin care

Introduction

When it comes to nappies you have a choice, and they are not mutually exclusive.

Disposable

More expensive, and arguably less friendly towards the environment, but very convenient. Some parts of the world take a dim view of paper nappies. There are horror stories of people trying to make disposable nappies last longer through re-use.

Re-usable

Just as all vacuum cleaners tend to be referred to as Hoovers, so re-usable nappies tend to be called Terries. They are cheaper, even with the cost of sterilising and washing. Probably kinder to the environment, but do require more work and a certain fatalism towards smells, especially from under the finger nails. You will need at least 20 as the inter-baby procedures take time.

Unlike disposable nappies which come pre-built, Terries are the 'flat pack' variety and need support systems such as:
- Nappy pins.
- Nappy liners. These can be disposable or re-usable.
- Plastic pants. Either elastic or tie-on. Tiny babies generally need the tie-on variety. Buy at least 5 pairs.
- Sterilising bucket plus fluid or powder.

Flat terries can be fastened with a product called a Nappy Nippa (a Y-shaped piece of thin rubber with claws on each end that grab the Terry). This avoids the risk of sticking a pin in your baby by accident. Many re-usables do up with poppers or with Velcro.

Changing nappies

Tools required
- Cotton wool roll.
- Changing mat. Preferably washable plastic (you will soon see why).
- Warm water/baby wipes. If your baby has any kind of rash or broken skin, using a baby wipe will soon turn them into a very angry octopus and twice as hard to get hold of. Think of aftershave on a sore chin.
- Barrier cream. This will help prevent nappy rash but cannot replace keeping the baby clean and changed often.
- A nappy tool box is useful for keeping all the above in (except the water).

How to do it
Disposable or otherwise there are some things you need to do which are common to both.

Remove nappy. If dirty set to one side for disposal/sterilising.

> Greasy fingers on the disposable nappy adhesive tabs renders them totally useless unless you have some insulating tape handy.

> When changing nappies (boy) always wear a waterproof hat or have an umbrella to hand.

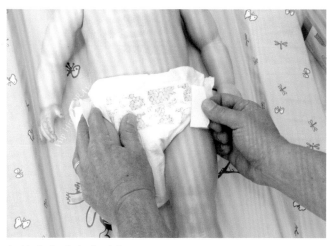

1 Undo the fastening tabs

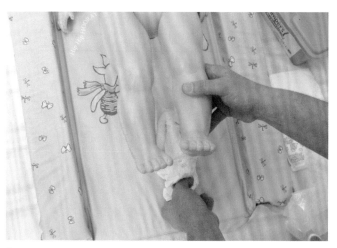

2 Lift up the baby and pull out the used nappy

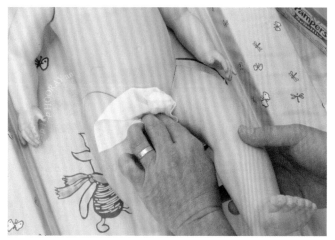

3 Clean the baby's bottom with warm water and cotton wool or with baby wipes

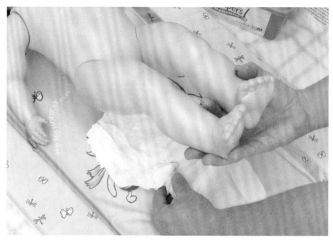

4 Slide the clean nappy underneath the baby. Make sure the nappy is the right way round

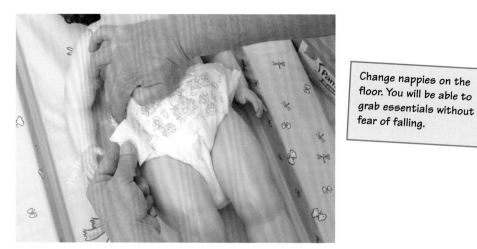

5 Bring the front of the nappy up through the baby's legs and fasten with the tabs

Change nappies on the floor. You will be able to grab essentials without fear of falling.

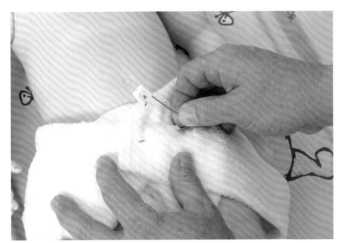

1 Remove the safety pin

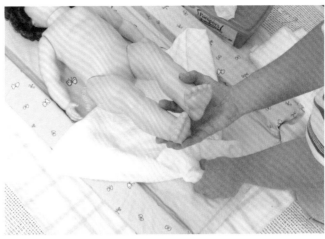

2 Lift up the baby and pull out the used nappy

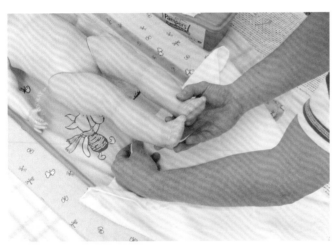

3 Clean the baby with warm water and cotton wool or baby wipes, then slide clean folded nappy underneath (see page 100 for kite fold)

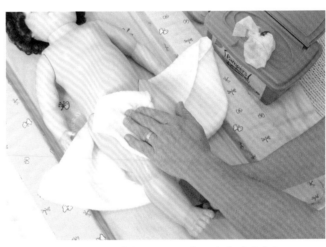

4 Bring the centre part of the nappy up through the baby's legs

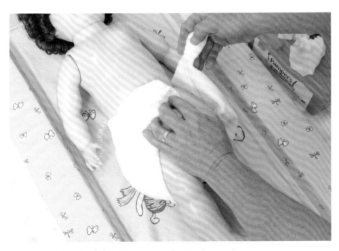

5 Fold the sides of the nappy over the centre part . . .

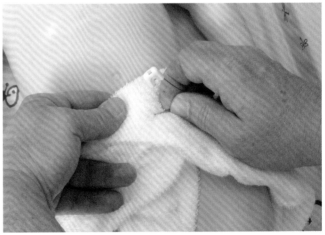

6 . . . and secure with a safety pin. Keep your fingers between the nappy and the baby so that if you make a mistake, you prick your finger and not the baby

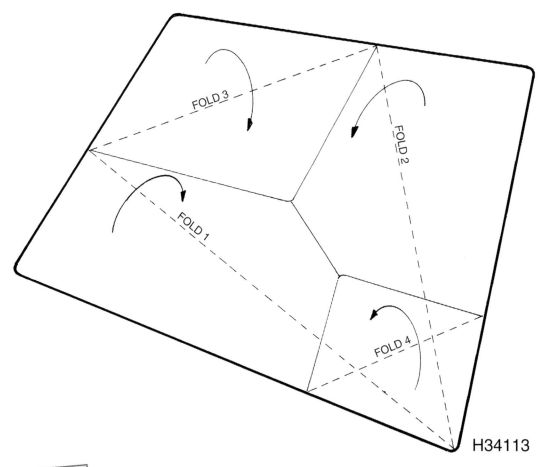

H34113

Folding a Terry nappy (kite fold)

Wash bottom with cotton wool and warm water and dry thoroughly. Some people advocate cleaning baby girls from front to back to prevent infection. Clean baby boy's foreskin but do not retract.

● Apply barrier cream (optional – regular changing is better).
● Avoid talcum powder.
● Fit nappy.
● Wash hands, sniff finger nails, wash hands again.

Things to watch out for

Expect big changes in the appearance and smell of their nappies as the child gets older.

Immediately after birth they will probably pass a green/black goo called meconium which is simply all the debris built up in the bowels during development in the womb.

As milk is increasingly digested you will see a yellow/orange colour. Breast-fed babies tend to have less solid motions than bottle fed. They also smell 'sweeter'. Like adults there is no 'normal' number of motions. None for more than a few days, or profuse watery motions, needs a doctor's attention (see *Diarrhoea* on page 151).

Stools can be so large you wonder how on earth they fitted in such a tiny body. Unfortunately they can cause small tears at the anus which makes passing subsequent motion very painful. Bright red blood streaked on the outside of the stool is common in these cases, but any blood in the motion must be reported to your doctor.

Also see *Nappy rash* on page 166)

Nappy contents colour chart

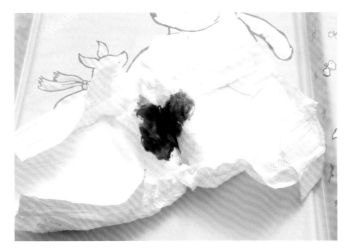

Green-black, sticky goo - meconium. Normal in new-born babies

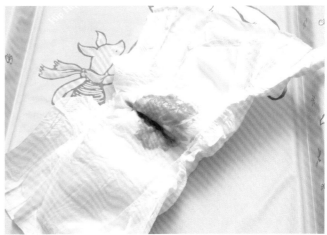

Yellow, loose - normal in breast-fed babies

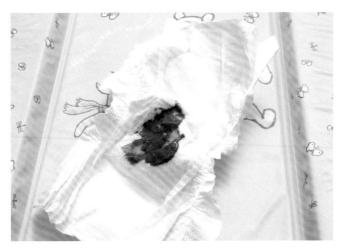

Orange, loose - also normal in breast-fed babies

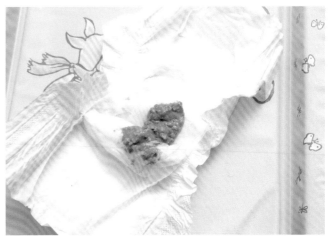

Orange, more solid - normal in bottle-fed babies

Green - sometimes normal, especially when changing from breast to bottle-feeding. Otherwise can be associated with colic

PART 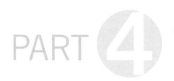 **Teething**

Introduction

Your baby's first teeth to appear will be the front incisors and they don't usually give much bother to the child in his or her first year. Although there is considerable variation between babies the times of teething average out as follows:

- 6 months first incisors (front teeth).
- 7 months second incisors.
- 12 months first molars.
- 18 months canines (eye teeth).
- 2-3 years second molars.
- Full set 20 teeth.

Symptoms

Inflammation of the gums with more dribbling than usual are generally accompanied by chewing fingers or anything else such as teething rings that comes along.

> When baby is teething, put chew toy in fridge to cool, when baby chews on the toy it numbs the pain in the gums.

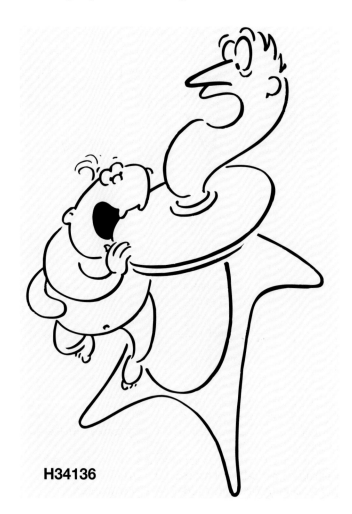

H34136

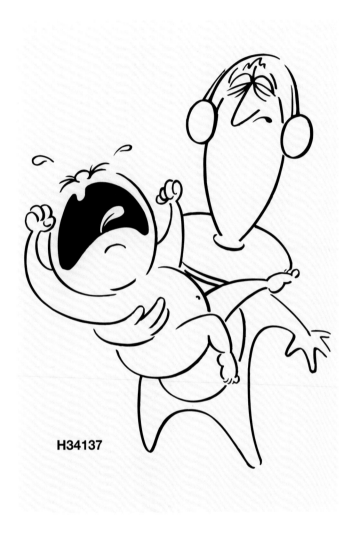

H34137

Causes

First and second molars (the back teeth) usually come through between 1 and 3 years of age and are much more likely to cause pain. Hot cheeks, tender gums and irritability are all common during this time.

Prevention

Letting them chew early can help.

Self help

Cool teething rings, cool drinks and gently rubbing the gums can all help. Excessive use of local anaesthetic gels is not helpful in the long run, as it is the action of chewing which allows the teeth to cut through.

Other conditions such as ear infections can be mistaken for teething. If your baby will not settle or has a high temperature you should ring NHS Direct (0845 46 47) or your GP.

PART 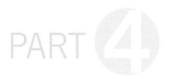 4

Talking and bonding

Introduction

Dads are people who give great hugs but are a bit short on the goodies, especially when it comes to breastfeeding. Babies have relatively little contact with their father in the early days. Awareness of there being two important people in their lives arrives slowly with time. Dads are usually waiting in the wings. Children become aware of their fathers gradually and some dads do the same thing with regard to their new baby.

It is a reflection of just how powerful a simple show of affection can be that as the child grows they are prepared, occasionally, to leave the arms of their source of food, their breastfeeding mother, for those of their father. Cuddle quality is important.

It's not all one-sided benefit either, having something to cuddle, even a cat or dog, prolongs life. This is supported by statistics which show that men in stable partnerships with children live longer on average than single men with no children.

Talking

For most men they say their relationship with their child really takes off once they start talking. Just as well, give the average man a 3 week old baby and all the efforts of parents and teachers to convey good English goes out with the nappy liner. It's not surprising that so much of language is rendered obsolete. Talking, if we mean communication, actually takes place very

> The secret to a good relationship with your child is to treat them as an adult that doesn't know anything. Intelligence starts high and reduces through life, the child will see through your lies, your incredible threats (if you don't stop that you won't get any Christmas presents...) and your faults and weaknesses. If you do something wrong have the guts to say you're sorry, otherwise you can never expect good behaviour from them. Look the child in the face when you talk, even the youngest baby. If they talk, stop and listen, even if you're busy. This gives them a sense of importance and self worth. If Mum and Dad don't value their opinions and thoughts why would anyone else?

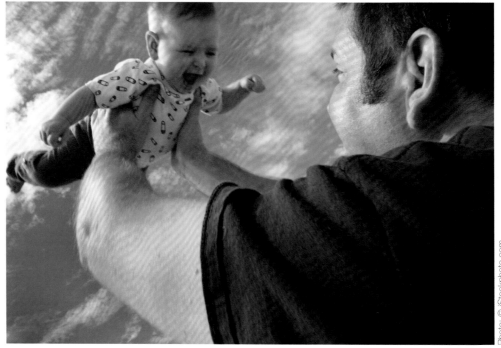

Photo: © iStockphoto.com

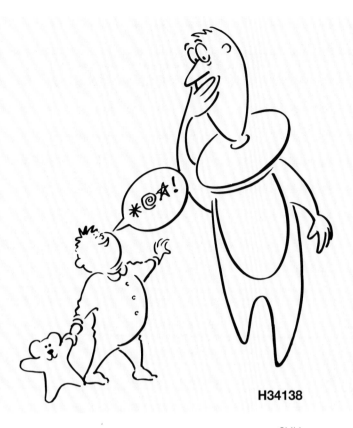

H34138

soon after birth. Babies indicate what they want very effectively by using their voice. Mothers can tell the often subtle difference between cries from the demand for food to that of wanting attention. Fathers are also able to do so, but usually later on. Conversation also takes place. Inflections in voice, along with the urgency with which it is spoken by the baby, convey a great deal of information. Some babies respond to loud talking, others to soft gentle speech. This may reflect the amount of 'background' noise in the home but may also be an expression of their own personality. From this type of contact we very quickly learn what babies like in the style of conversation. Admittedly much of the conversation is one way.

Fashion changes between generations on the style which should be used when speaking to a baby. Modernists reject 'baby talk' and insist that we speak to them as miniature adults. Traditionalists say this is useless and robs the child of the intimacy of such talk. Much of 'love talk' between adults would fail a test of good English. Eye contact is maintained with changes in tonal inflection of speech. Speech of whatever form which maintains a constant pitch does not have the same attraction to babies. Rhetoric is probably appreciated at a very early age and as all politicians know well, on occasion it is not what you say that counts, but how you say it.

All babies probably get a mixture of both as they are constantly picking up conversation not directed to themselves. Children suddenly repeat a phrase or word which most certainly would not have been meant for their ears. With exquisite timing, they will always wait until they are in the most genteel company of adoring aunts before making these utterances. Babies adore repetition, especially in speech. Telling or singing the same nursery rhyme may be boring to you, but to your baby it is a recognisable pattern in an otherwise chaotic world. Even as they

Children are constantly picking up conversation not directed at themselves . . .

grow older the desire for repeatability remains and reading the same story over again becomes par for the course. Children will allow a certain amount of variation on the theme but the basic structure has to remain the same. It is the gentle nuances in speech which introduce variation. Not a million miles away from constantly sung football or rugby songs, adult men find security in the predictable chant as do their children. It is the group involvement which supplies the confidence. Singing a nursery rhyme, for the 100th time conveys commitment and security. Experimentation is the name of the game, so long as it is within certain boundaries of familiarity.

His father's voice

Babies are already exposed to their mother's speech while in the womb. This is reinforced by intimate contact after being born. Babies are often little disturbed by a mother's sneeze or cough. Men have not only traditionally been slow to talk to their babies, possibly through self-consciousness, but they have had less opportunity to do so. Many men leave for work while their children are in bed and return from work to find them in the same place. Despite the changes which are taking place in work patterns, men in the UK still work the longest hours in the EU. For all these reasons, and more besides, the baby learns and becomes accustomed to dad's voice after mum's. Get your face in there as well. If your baby can't recognise your mug shot they will cry, which just puts you off trying in the first place.

Just point

Frustration is written all over the face of a child who can understand speech but whose brain has not yet worked out how to actually speak. A similar but more devastating phenomenon occurs with the adult brain which has been damaged by stroke. A common result of such injury is the ability of the person to recognise an object but be unable to state its name. A watch becomes 'time' or 'day'. Such is the frustration they will often substitute a string of expletives which can be startling in their clarity compared to the hesitant inaccurate speech of which they

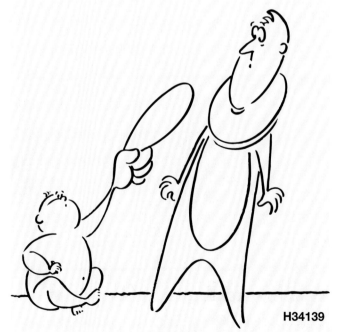

The pointing finger is a powerful tool

H34139

are normally capable. Babies and toddlers are just as frustrated and will become impatient when you fail to understand that the unintelligible collection of consonants they are hurling at you at top volume simply means 'I want a biscuit'. Interestingly, they will often treat the adult as an idiot and turn to one of their older siblings to act as an interpreter who promptly says, with just a touch of superiority, 'He wants a biscuit daddy'. When all else fails on the language front, babies will simply point a finger until you get it right. This can lead to a crescendo of frustration both from the baby, who patently considers the father an idiot, and the father who simply feels like an idiot. Part of the pleasure of fatherhood is getting the pointing finger correct and being able to say the noun of the object of desire. Like many facets of parenthood it is usually short-lived as your baby recognises a way of maintaining attention even when there is no immediate object of desire. The pointing finger is truly a powerful tool in learning the name of things and keeping you there.

Experimenting with speech

Their ability to experiment with words and language will is vital for coping with many other facets of learning later on in their development. Some dads find talking to a baby very difficult. Often these dads will also find small-talk difficult, and would prefer to say nothing rather than talk just for the sake of it. If you are like this, and you are in the majority of dads, look for opportunities to chat.

Dressing

Babies and toddlers are fascinated by clothes. It also helps you if you 'talk them down' through all the various bits. The same thing happens when putting them back on again. Baby-gros can produce a most stimulating conversation, as there always appears to be one press-stud too many; now is the time to practice expletive-free conversation. Feeding is a similar opportunity for conversation, you won't be the first father to explain that the rapidly approaching spoonful of baby food is in fact a train about to enter a tunnel.

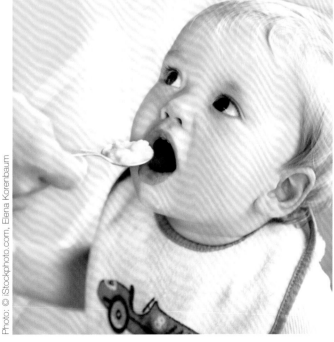

Photo: © iStockphoto.com, Elena Korenbaum

Picture books

A time-honoured way of promoting interaction. You supply the commentary and pointing finger, they supply the laughs and impatience to see the next page even though you are only half-way through this one. Don't underestimate what is going in during these sessions. Many a baby will let you know very quickly if you have turned the page before they have digested the previous one completely. Memory in a young child is uncluttered with telephone numbers, useless facts and dates. They have plenty of room, therefore, for what you said the last time you went through a particular story. Going too fast and skipping large chunks will be noticed by your child, who will not be slow to let you know what they think of the room service.

Question-time

Conversations should be two way. Asking questions like 'Did you like that?' may not produce definitive answers but you may be rewarded by a gleeful shout. Remember to answer their questions as well. They may not sound like questions but any response is

better than none. Avoid answering your own questions too often and allow them time to make their verbal or non-verbal response.

Milestones of development

Being involved as a father is not only important to your child, it is important for your memories of how they grew up. The fun comes from listening out for the stages of language development. A mixture of pleasure and fear, listening to a child experiment with words raises apprehension over the speed of their development. Medical text books will lay down milestones through which the child should pass during normal development. These indicators of 'normal' development can be a source of constant worry for the parents of completely normal children who fail to meet the deadline on time. Failure to build a tower of four bricks can be endured but a failure to talk is often seen as a real disaster and portends failure in society. If these books are read carefully they will explain that 'normality' is not only impossible to define but that it is also undesirable when talking about human beings of whatever age.

Most doctors happily settle for the average age at which a milestone will be reached with the sure knowledge that there will be children who are a little above or below this average yet will be as 'normal' as the next child. Teachers and health visitors are probably better people to talk to than doctors and they will agree with the medical profession that children have different rates of development in different areas. One of our children was slow to perfect their speech and was borderline for help from the speech therapist. More important was that she could experiment with language and would use it to produce the greatest response for her demands rather than praise for grammatical correctness. Your health visitor can check on their speed of development.

Silence can be golden

Allow some mistakes in their speech. Constant correction will impede experimentation. Nursery rhymes, songs and chants are all good ways of instilling confidence in a child in the use of language and do not need to be in BBC English. Patience and encouragement will pay great dividends when your child first tries to tell a story, and will allow them to develop their expression through language. Energetic use of language to get a message across, which is why it was invented in the first place, is more important in the early stages than its grammatical accuracy. Exactly when they start is less important than how. If a child can get by with expressions and body language easily interpreted by their brothers or sisters, it may reduce the stimulus for talking. Alternatively, the intimate and often sustained contact with their brothers and sisters who are talking, increases the exposure to speech. All our children began to speak at different times and it had little if any effect on their ability at school.

Phonetic Phun

We tend to enforce our cultural speech on their first words. A bottle can become a bo bo. A similar and long-standing teaching method occurs with phonetic teaching where letters of the

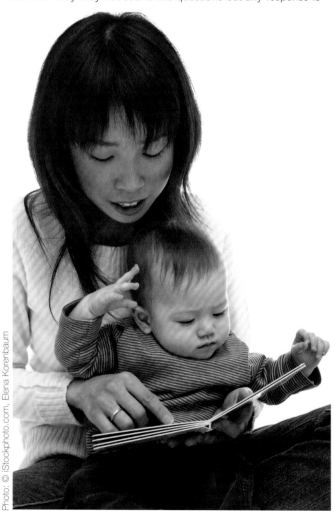

Photo: © iStockphoto.com, Elena Korenbaum

Keep a bag of toys and books permanently in the car. If you can stretch to it, buy duplicates of a few small toys so that you can have one set permanently in the car and one set at home.

alphabet take on their phonetic sounds. Ah, Buh, Cuh, etc, can be considered an extension of the baby talk which was once called 'mother tongue'. Part of the fun of having children is their use of grammatically incorrect language giving us all a chuckle. Like Father Christmas and Peter Pan, it may be part of a desire to preserve the state of childhood for as long as possible.

Play

Play is the great leveller, bringing both baby and father to the same plane of simply having fun. Without doubt there may be an unconscious attempt to teach and learn, but as a bond, for a brief spell, baby and father are united in warmth and need no language. Given that play appears to have no constructive value it tends to be delegated to people who 'have more free time'. This is the equivalent of growing a prize melon but letting someone else eat it. Play is a learning experience. It not only develops ability at art or construction, it also builds confidence, promotes sharing and even allows children to teach other children without them realising what they are doing. More important for fathers, it is a tax-free way of blowing off steam, doing something just because it is fun. Paradoxically, play with your child can be hard work. Even so there are ways of limiting the effort and increasing the pleasure.

Stories and plays
Children love stories and plays. It is part of getting ready for real life. They particularly like to act out what they hear and make up.

Puppets, and these can be as simple as socks or ice-lolly sticks tied together, provide a material basis for their imagination. Older children tend to direct; like the younger ones, you should be content to supply ideas and be the bad guy.

Painting
Painting comes naturally when young. Unfortunately young people tend to paint everything except the paper. Getting upset over the mess is about as useful as Canute opposing the next tide. Invest in a large sheet of plastic floor covering and sacks of brushes, paint and child-safe felt-tip pens. Avoid invoking rules for play with very young children. They will develop their own rules, which like politicians' oaths, tend to be flexible.

Imagination
Story-telling need not be straight from a book. Develop a theme such as 'islands to be ship-wrecked on', or 'tunnels that lead to...'. You only need to provide the canvas, they will supply the paint. Imagination is more powerful than any printer's ink.

The force of gravity
Children, like Newtonian apples, will always return to Earth. Children, however, have yet to be taught this basic fact of physics and consider it quite normal to be attached to their father's anatomy even when he is trying to use the toilet. Most men very soon realise that it is always easier to sit down rather than try the single-handed approach. As they slip inexorably lower down mum, they would be stopped by a hip, mum's hod-carrier.

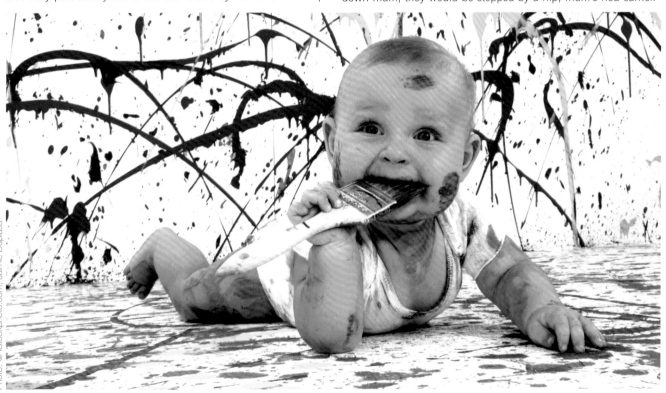

Photo: © iStockphoto.com, Jaimie Duplass

Unfortunately for men, nothing can halt this downward slide until a little heap of person is clutching a pair of knees. Dads are perceived, rightly or wrongly, as being stronger and you will often get away with more 'rough' play than your partner. Allowing them to ride around on your foot, having slipped all the way down from your chest, may not be particularly comfortable, but it is awesome to a child and probably stops your blood vessels furring up.

Feeding

Eating is not the same as feeding. Babies feed, they do not eat. This is not to say they do not appreciate good taste. What defines 'good taste' to a baby may have a great deal to do with texture. The difference has nothing to do with what is eaten, but rather, how it is eaten. Babies approach this by the two steps forward, one step back method.

If bottle feeding, it is important to follow the instructions on the tin very carefully. It is not simply because of the amount which may or may not be taken, although this is important to make sure the baby has enough food, but also to maintain the dilution of the food with water. If it is too concentrated the baby will become constipated and may even become dehydrated. Too dilute and the baby will be constantly hungry and will pass very loose motions.

To cure constipation simply remove nappy.

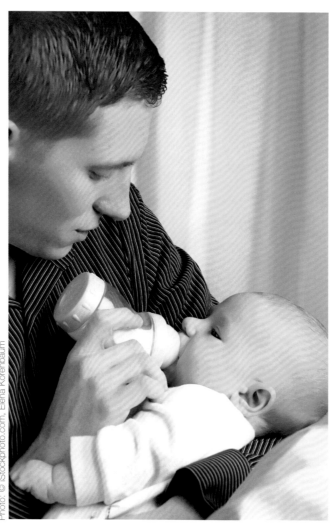

Photo: © iStockphoto.com, Elena Korenbaum

Gastroenteritis is uncommon in breast-fed babies. Very young babies rely to large extent upon the natural defences against infection passed on from the mother during pregnancy and from breast milk. Bottles and teats, therefore, need to be kept as clean as possible by the use of sterilising agents.

Every father will find his own method of feeding which works for him. Some form of gentle distraction such as rocking or background music can help. I personally exhausted my entire memory of Beatles songs which, along with a bit of rock-and-roll, seemed to do the trick.

Vomiting comes with the feeding. It is normal for the baby to bring up a fair proportion of what went down.

Warning signs

It is the failure to feed, or the irritation during feeding, which should set off alarm bells. Babies have a very limited reserve of fluid and will dehydrate quickly if they are vomiting repeatedly or have profuse diarrhoea. Skin which remains puckered when gently pinched between thumb and finger can be a sign of dehydration.

Repeated vomiting, particularly if followed by a demand for more food, may be a sign of a very treatable condition of pyloric stenosis. It involves a progressive narrowing of the opening of the stomach and is characterised by repeated vomiting in the very young baby. This type of vomiting is hard to miss as it is highly projectile and will travel a metre or so across the floor. Babies with this condition rapidly lose weight but with early recognition of the problem will rarely come to any harm.

Bonding through feeding

To feed a person, baby or otherwise, establishes a bond, the significance of which is never lost between both parties. Watching someone eat and enjoy their food is part of human contact and is the basis of many 'food' programmes on the TV. Many chefs, male and female, will admit that they enjoy preparing food and watching other people eat more than eating the food themselves. Watching your own child feed is even more special and you will be assured of 'many happy returns'. While breastfeeding is without doubt the best way, it does tend to marginalise the dad. A father's time will come, however, and food from dad's plate always tastes better than their own.

What is important from these intimacies is not just the ability to talk, feed or play. It is the effect each has on the bond which develops between a very young person and an older one. Fathers have an uphill struggle against what is expected of them. A steep learning curve is involved with little to go on except what has been traditionally performed by mothers. Innovation is the key as we have everything to gain from experimentation.

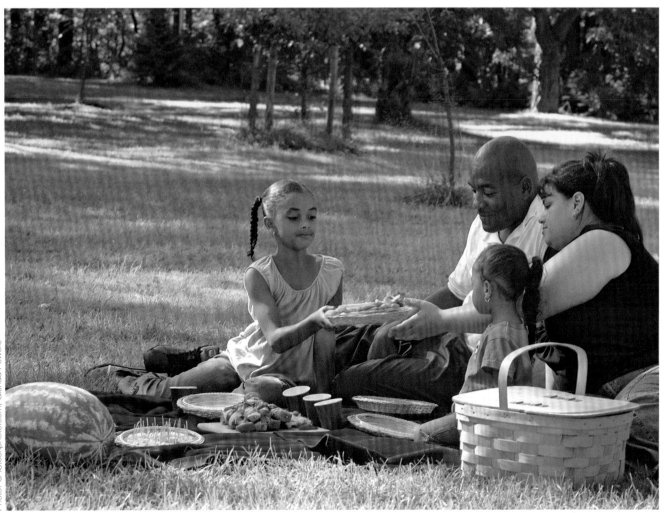

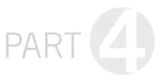

Shopping

Introduction

Fathers increasingly take their children shopping and also increasingly complain of having nowhere to take their new baby when they need a fresh nappy. It's worth contacting stores before hand to find out about their facilities. Some men were using the toilets intended for disabled people as they often contain changing mats for babies. Thankfully things are changing.

> I always found a paper bag, commonly used for putting mushrooms in, would keep my son amused whilst I was doing my shopping because of the noise it made.

Advances in shopping

As society's expectation of men as fathers changes it is becoming common not only to see men with prams and buggies but also to see them doing the shopping for the family, along with their young baby, in supermarkets. It can be easy to run away with the idea that supermarkets are all run by managers who just love children. If they are, they only demonstrated their affection after the effects of competition began to bite into their profits. Hard discounters are taken very seriously by the supermarket chains and they cannot compete except on service. Thus the sudden change of heart. Most chains now advertise the pleasure their store is for a family. With all the changes that are taking place, to make your shopping life as easy as possible, it makes sense to phone around first. The message will not be lost on the managers as the number of calls increase.

Parking

One of the nightmares for a parent is the availability of car parking spaces. Shopping means negotiating an obstacle course of speeding cars driven by frustrated drivers intent on leaving the area as soon as humanly possible; trolley parks that require a mint condition pound piece and are the furthest distance away from the last remaining car park space; bollards to prevent trolleys wandering but would double admirably as tank traps, and spaces so narrow that parking a car full of children means at least a respray after they open the doors. Parking dedicated to parents with children, close to the entrance, such as exists for disabled drivers, makes sense and is beginning to appear.

Access

While it may make sense to pack every square millimetre with sellable goods, the narrow isle is asking for the 'Royal Mail Train Effect'. Anyone who has watched a train pick up a mail bag while on the move will recognise the analogy when taking a trolley loaded with children down a supermarket isle. It is at this point that the analogy ends. While the mail bag invariably arrives safely on board the speeding train, the extra large bottle of tomato ketchup ends its life as a spectacular pool on the floor.

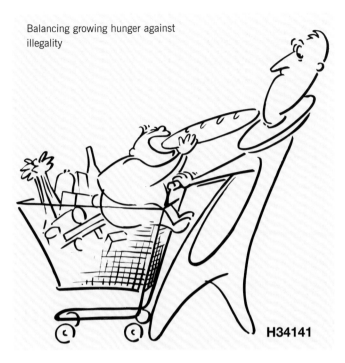

Balancing growing hunger against illegality

H34141

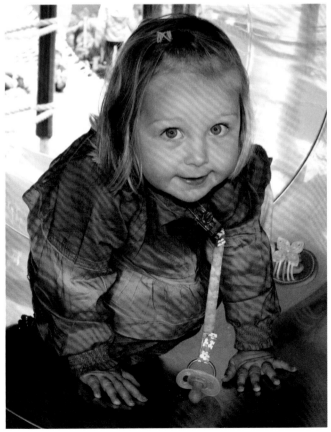

Trolleys

Supermarkets appear to believe that families consist of one child. Furthermore, the trolley is designed for a baby which can sit, unaided, in a metal framework which is ergometrically sound for folding away but has little to do with safety. A range of trolleys makes sense and is being introduced into the larger stores.

Corridor of hell, the checkout

Waiting with children at a checkout bedecked with sweets is not just a dentist's nightmare. Look out for stores which have extra staff at checkouts to help with the packing. They have been trained to 'home in' on the customers with a crying or difficult child.

Changing-rooms and toilets

Given the shift towards buying in bulk for a family, the time spent in a supermarket can be considerable. Children have small bladders, babies need to be changed. For men this presents two problems, finding a toilet and finding a toilet which caters for men to look after their children. While there has been recent improvement, some supermarkets have changing rooms only for mothers with the helpful provision that 'staff will find room for fathers'. If ever there was a feeling of being the second class citizen, having 'staff finding room' for you must be a major contributor.

Eating

Just as children's bladders are small, so are their stomachs. At some point children will balance their growing hunger against the illegality of ripping the nearest packet of biscuits open. Given the strength of the instinct for human survival, it takes little imagination to picture the scene of chaos. Having the facilities for eating is not the same as facilitating for children. Most fast-food outlets have a limited menu for children and welcome them. Some will lay on special treats for birthdays. Restaurants are not usually so keen but will still have a special children's menu. Ask for a smaller sized adult meal or one between three - it is usually supplied with good grace and offers a better choice than the usual children's menu of chicken nuggets, fish fingers, chips ands baked beans.

Crèche facilities

Obviously the answer to shopping with children is the same as working with children. Get someone else to look after them while you shop. You can only play on the sympathy of the next door neighbour or relative for so long. Some supermarkets have introduced crèche facilities which allow you, for a small fee, to get on with the job. Play areas are not quite the same thing but some of them are supervised. With the increased fear of abduction, it makes good sense to insist upon supervised care.

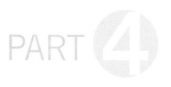

Baby problems

Introduction

Traditionally, women have taken on the role of 'home doctor'. Part of the reason why women present to their GP more often is the simple fact that they usually are 'deemed' responsible for bringing the children when they are ill or for vaccinations. Most medical education is directed towards women and mothers, particularly regarding very young children and babies. Men as fathers were less likely to ask for medical advice. This had more to do with society's expectation and the perception of the 'male role' than sound medical knowledge.

Objectivity can be difficult when you are suddenly responsible for the welfare of your child. While there is an army of people at the hospital, all dedicated to the health of your baby, at home you will be the link between your baby and this medical advice and help. Having knowledge is as important as being confident.

Small baby, but big changes

Temperature control is particularly poor, not least because of a baby's small body mass and relatively large surface area. Thus staying warm, or (possibly more importantly) staying cool, is not as easy as for an adult. During the settling period the baby may display all kinds of colour changes, spots, blotches, swellings and secretions. Thankfully, most of these changes are completely normal but can often look quite worrying. It is important to remember that when things do go wrong in a baby they tend to happen much faster than in an adult so if you are not sure about whether there is something really amiss, call NHS Direct (0845 46 47) or give your doctor a call. There may be nothing to worry about, but you will be reassured.

Peculiar shape head

All babies' heads are a strange shape when born. The skull bones are not completely joined together until 18 months or so after being born. This is to allow the baby's head to pass through the birth canal and in doing so it is invariably squeezed out of shape. Marks from forceps, particularly around the ears, are common and rarely cause any problems for long. Similarly, if your baby was delivered using the Ventouse cup there may be a 'cap' over the head which is caused by the suction of the cup. It will disappear slowly without harm. Babies who have been looked after in an incubator for a number of weeks tend to develop long heads, flattened at the sides. This is also temporary and will gradually disappear as your baby is able to move their head more freely.

Soft spots in the skull (fontanelles)

As the baby's head has not finished growing and the bones of the skull are not all joined together, there are two soft spots on the skull which have no bone beneath the skin. Many parents are unnecessarily scared to even touch these areas. In fact there is a very tough, thick membrane protecting these gaps in the bone and it is highly unlikely that normal handling will cause any harm. They can be very useful for checking if the baby is dehydrated as they will sink down with lack of water. If they are ever very taut or raised like small mounds, it can be a sign of illness. They do tend to do this if the baby is crying very hard, but will subside when the baby calms down. If they remain taut or distended you should call your doctor (see *Meningitis* on page 181)

Scurf on the scalp (cradle cap)

This is normal. It is not caused by a lack of hygiene. A really thick cap-shaped layer is called cradle cap. Remove it by gently rubbing with olive oil. There are lotions available from the chemist under prescription but as cradle cap is not harmful it is best left alone and it will settle of its own accord (see *Cradle cap* on page 164).

Hair

There is a great deal of ignorance and superstition over hair on a baby. In fact, any amount of hair on the head, from baldness to long flowing hair which reaches down the back, is normal. Extra time spent in the womb, say a couple of weeks, can often result in more hair. Most of the hair will be lost soon after birth anyway.

Eyes

No matter what colour you or your partner's eyes happen to be, most babies' eyes are blue at birth and they change colour gradually to that which will remain for the rest of their lives. Thankfully, the serious eye problems which were once associated with childbirth and are still seen in many underdeveloped countries, are now very uncommon in the UK.

Crusting on lids and lashes can be yellow and may even stick the lids together. This is normally the result of a very common mild infection known as sticky eye. It is not serious but the baby should be seen by the doctor who will recommend drops or a solution for bathing the eyes. Remove the crust using cotton wool soaked in water or saline (see *Sticky eye* on page 173).

Wandering eye: an eye which appears to have a mind of its own and wanders about, particularly when the baby is looking intently at something close up, is in most cases completely normal. If this persists, or if your baby can never appear to focus both eyes at the same time on an object, you should inform your doctor or health visitor.

Skin

A new baby's skin is delicious to kiss. They have a fragrance and softness which must have some effect on the adult smell and brain which enhances the protective instinct. Unfortunately their skin is easily damaged by their own urine, causing a nappy rash, and tight clothing or nappies which can tear the skin. Loose clothing, which presents no danger of suffocation, along with changing nappies before the skin reddens, will avoid most of these problems. New babies can also demonstrate an almost chameleon-like change of colour which can be alarming to watch yet rarely has any significance (see *Nappy rash* on page 166).

Spots and patches

The most common type of spots seen on new babies are red spots with yellow centres called neonatal urticaria. A big word for a small baby. These spots form because the baby's skin and its pores do not yet work efficiently. No treatment is required and they will invariably disappear after the first couple of weeks. Spots which look like bruises and do not turn white when you run your nail over them, especially if the baby is crying, off feeds, hot, or irritable, should be reported to your doctor as some forms of meningitis present in this fashion. Generally speaking, however, if the baby is feeding, appears happy and is not crying, is not increasingly drowsy and has a normal temperature, a spot does not mean a lot.

Ear wax and smelly discharge

All babies will have wax in their ears. While it is reasonable to remove any wax which appears at the very outside of the ear, trying to remove wax from within the ear will only result in packing the wax in tighter and irritate the ear canal such that it will produce even more wax. A smelly discharge, often yellow in colour, particularly if the baby is irritable, may indicate an infection. Your doctor can advise.

Swelling abdomen

Many babies will have a swelling just around the navel. It will be more pronounced when they cry or pass a motion. It is caused by a weakness in the muscle in the area of the navel which originally allowed blood to flow through the umbilical cord. Although it is called an umbilical hernia most right themselves completely by one year. Very few ever require surgery, which if it is required is a very simple operation performed when the child is a bit older. If your baby has a permanently distended abdomen, particularly if they are not passing any motions and are vomiting repeatedly, you should inform your doctor (see *Crying baby* on page 185).

Vomiting

Posseting of a little milk after feeds is normal. Repeated vomiting, particularly if the vomiting is so violent that the vomit travels a half metre or so (projectile vomiting) needs the attention of your doctor as there could be an obstruction in the stomach or bowel. Fortunately such obstructions are now readily treatable by a relatively simple operation (see *Vomiting in babies* on page 153).

Crying

The only way a baby can communicate to you that they are not happy is by crying. It may not be the most informative way of telling you what they want but there is usually a pattern in the cry which most mothers, and increasingly fathers, can interpret as being either minor, important or requires urgent action. Generally speaking, if it is possible to distract them with a cuddle or play, then it is not serious. If they continue to cry despite your very best attempts with aeroplanes, trains, noises from the jungle and old-fashioned cuddles, then it may be because of:

● **A dirty nappy**. Never underestimate the effect of urine in contact with raw skin. A child who cries and then stops when the nappy has been changed has given you their verdict (see *Nappy rash* on page 166).

● **Lack of food**. Hunger is a powerful stimulus for a baby to cry. How else will they make clear that it is time to feed? Nature has ensured that this type of cry is particularly piercing, persistent and difficult to ignore. Small bodies need small amounts of food but regularly. Night is the same as day to a small stomach. Babies who continue to cry even when being fed are trying to tell you something. Feeding is a natural analgesic and comforter, but if the real cause of the crying is not hunger, and if your baby is not settled by feeding, look for another possible cause.

● **Windy stomach or colic**. A build-up of gas in the bowel, which is common when your sole source of food is milk, can cause pressure on the bowel and thus pain. It will also stop you from taking any more food even though you are hungry. Net result, a spasmodic cry which is often relieved by simply changing the position of the baby with gentle tapping. A sudden release of pressure from either end, followed by a cessation of crying, gives you your answer. There are medications available for babies who are particularly prone to wind and colic, but as most cases of wind and colic are self-limiting, they are best avoided until all the simple, time-honoured methods such as rhythmic movement have been tried and exhausted, like yourself (see *Abdominal pain* on page 150).

● **Hot, cold, lonely, sleepy, fed up**. As a baby cannot move to somewhere better, they can only cry to make things better for themselves where they are at that particular moment. If they are too hot, cold or fed up with staring at the same ceiling for two hours, they may cry. Similarly, and paradoxically, if they are sleepy they may also cry. Recognising the pattern of the cry is important but at the end of the day, and it usually is, you may not be able to identify just what is really wrong other than that it is nothing serious.

Although the majority of babies do not cry continuously, crying can cause considerable exhaustion in parents. This is true for both you and your partner, and may cause friction in your relationship, particularly as men still do not have the legal right to remain at home during much of this exciting but demanding period. Some babies cry more than others, even within the same family. After trying all the stand-bys, soothers, rocking, music, singing and dancing you need to take a break. If there is obviously nothing serious, step back for a while. It will not hurt to let your baby cry on for a few minutes while you have a cup of tea and rest. Taking turns between you and your partner helps give each other a break. Often your return and a fresh approach will do the trick. Talking to others about it can help. You may be surprised at how many people have lived through the same experience. The name of the game is to pace yourself. An exhausted father with an exhausted baby is not a good combination, spread the load if possible.

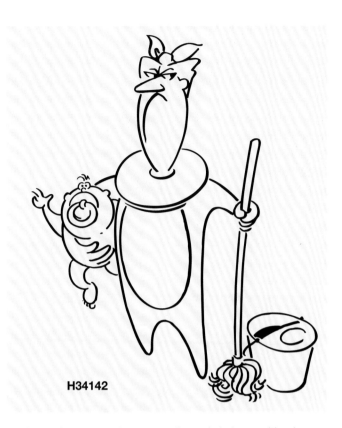

H34142

If there is a change in pattern of your baby's cry, either in duration, nature or sound, it may mean there is a problem. Every now and then check that none of the other causes of crying have returned to prolong the agony. Keep your mind open to a real problem if your baby never normally cries in this way (see *Crying baby* on page 185).

Bed-time and lack of sleep

For very young babies the 24 hour day is broken up into periods of sleep, awake and feeding. Night-time is not a concept with which they have yet become acquainted. Some babies will sleep longer than others. Similarly, some babies will feed longer than others. You will find ways of improving the sleep pattern of your baby. For instance an absolutely quiet house may well help to maintain their sleep, but as this is almost impossible, it is a good idea to get them accustomed to ordinary house-hold noise while they sleep. A warm bath or feed just before putting them to bed can also help.

Sleep deprivation is a well-recognised form of torture. It can disrupt your normal life, relationship with your partner and sour the enjoyment a new baby should bring. If it is possible, allow each other to share the load. It is desirable, but obviously not always possible, to allow your partner to nap during the day if she is breastfeeding. Bottle feeding, whether from expressed milk or concentrate, obviously will allow you to take part of the responsibility for night feeds. Even in the mind fogged, sleep deprived fugue it helps to know that this period of mixed torment with pleasure, will not last so long. Until the next child comes along, that is. Strangely, you tend to forget the bad bits and remember only the feeling of peace and exhilaration of holding a new baby when the decision whether or not to increase the size of the family comes around.

Some babies go to sleep more easily if they are swaddled fairly tightly. Try rocking them in your arms and making loud 'shhh' noises.

If your young child won't go to sleep, take them out for a drive in the car (even in the wee small hours - although your neighbours may think you're mad!) - it will often send them off to sleep, and you can drive them home and pop them into bed. A walk in the pram will often do the same thing.

PART 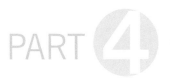 Child development

Contrary to constant desire for standardisation, there is no such thing as 'normal development'. In terms of weight gain, behavioural changes, speech and walking there are only averages and all children develop at different rates, attaining skills at different ages. Being 'slow' to walk is not a sign of poor development. Similarly 'delayed' speech is not a sign of impaired intellect. You should consider all the various milestones and discuss them with your health visitor.

Newly born

Movement and posture.

- Running your finger across the palms causes a 'grasp' reaction (the baby grips your finger).
- Lifting the baby up by the arms from the lying position to the sitting position, the head lags behind.
- When your baby's body is held face down, the head droops, the legs hang down and arms are flexed.
- If placed face down, the head turns to the side, the legs are flexed under the body and arms are held close in with elbows bent.

Eyes and responses.

- The baby's pupils react to light and it closes its eyes to sudden brightness. It opens its eyes when lifted upright.

One month

Movement and posture.

- When the sole of the foot is stimulated or tickled, the baby bends its leg up at the knee as if to pull it away.
- When lying on its back, the baby turns its head to one side and stretches out its arm and leg on that side.
- When active, both arms and legs make large jerky movements but when still, the fists are usually closed with the thumb turned in.
- If you touch the corner of its mouth the baby turns its head towards that side to suck, but when its ear is touched, it turns its head away.
- The baby's head still lags when it is lifted by its arms to the sitting position.
- The baby makes 'walking' movements with legs when held by the body over a surface.

Eyes and responses.

- Eyes will follow its mother's face.
- May blink on sudden movement near its face.
- Shows interest by staring at a window or bright colours.
- Turns its head towards light and shuts its eyes in sudden bright light.

Play.

- Begins to respond by moving its arms and legs while being dressed and bathed and makes noises in response to being spoken to.
- Begins to smile at around six weeks and stops crying when picked up and spoken to unless something is wrong.

Six months

Movement and posture.

- Tries to sit when hands are held and may even sit upright for a few seconds.
- Seeks being picked up and holds its arms out for cuddles.
- Can lift its legs and grasp them with its hands, occasionally attempting to suck a toe.
- If laid on its back, the baby will lift up its head off the surface and sit up with support and move its arms purposefully.
- Will stand if held on a hard surface, attempting to bounce up and down.

Eyes and responses.

- Can hold a toy and moves it from hand to hand.
- Will respond to objects seen out of the corner of its eye. It is now very interested in its surroundings and moves its head often. Follows parents' movements for long periods of time.
- Squints, if present, should now be gone and if present should be referred to a doctor.
- If toy falls out of sight, forgets it.

Play.

- Will put everything to its mouth and will reach for a rattle and suck it when holding it.
- Will examines objects attentively, often moving from hand to hand.
- Now beginning to become reserved with strangers.

Speech.

- Can recognise mother's voice immediately and makes singing noises when content.
- Now learnt to laugh and squeals loudly when pleased but screams when annoyed.
- Can understand different tones of mother's voice.

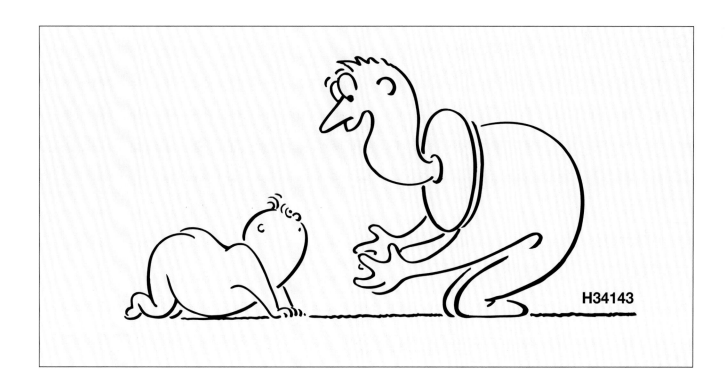

H34143

One year

Movement and posture.
- May stand alone for a few seconds and may walk with assistance.
- Can sit itself up from lying down and will sit for indefinite periods on the floor playing happily
- Will crawl on hands and knees and can move quite rapidly.
- Is fully able to pull itself to a standing position and lay itself down again.

Eyes and responses.
- Now holding an object in each hand, knocking them together.
- Drops and throws deliberately to see what happens and points at wanted objects.
- Often recognises known faces the other side of the room.
- Possibly able to show preference in using right or left hand.

Play.
- Shows pleasure in seeing familiar faces.
- Finds toys if they are totally hidden while it is watching.
- Prefers and seeks toys that make a sound.
- Hands toys to parents and release them by opening the hand.
- Plays pat-a-cake and waves bye-bye.
- Drinks well from normal cup and will hold out arms and legs for dressing.
- Tries to ring toy bell by shaking it if shown how to do it.

Speech.
- Speech-like sounds taking inflection and form.
- Parents will be able to recognise from 2 to 6 words that the baby says.
- Can understand simple instruction like, 'Give it to Mummy.'
- Knows and responds to own name.
- Understands a number of words, such as ball, cup and spoon.

18 months

Movement and posture.
- Often carries a favourite toy such as a teddy bear by an arm or leg.
- Now walks upstairs with assistance, but not downstairs.
- Now playing and picking up toys.
- Might walk alone, both starting and stopping without falling and may run, but is stopped by obstacles.

Eyes and responses.
- Finger grasp now more subtle, can pick up pins and can hold a pencil quite simply.
- Points at distant objects.
- Turning pages of a book.
- Recognises previously seen books and contents.
- Builds a tower of 3 cubes.

Speech.
- Can now use and understand around 20 words and enjoys nursery rhymes.
- Understands and will point to hair, nose, feet and hands.
- Likes singing.
- 'Talks' loudly and continuously while playing.
- Will follow spoken instructions.

2 years 6 months

Eyes and responses.

- Recognises a picture of self.
- Attentive to small detail in pictures.
- Can build a tower of 10 cubes using one hand and can usually draw a circle.

Play.

- May watch other children play but not necessarily join in.
- May throw a tantrum when restrained.
- Playing for long periods with toys but still requires parents' attention.
- Eating and drinking successfully with spoon and is usually dry through night and can pull down pants for toilet.

Motorway service cafeterias are good places to start teaching your children how to feed themselves. Clearing up the high chair and the surrounding floor is someone else's job.

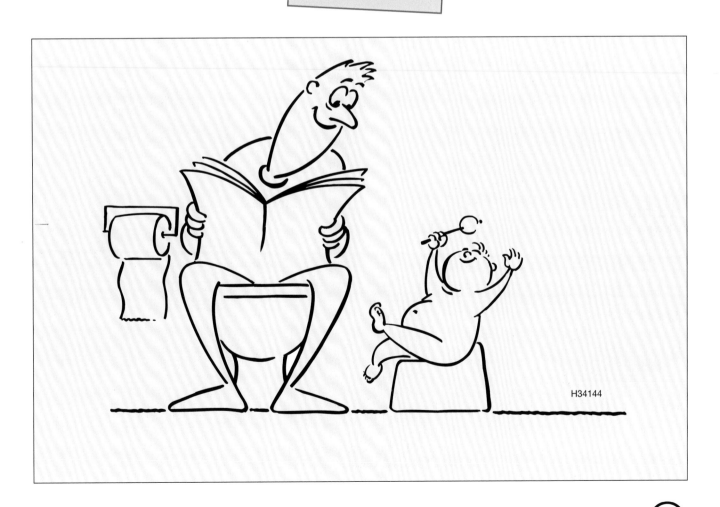

H34144

5

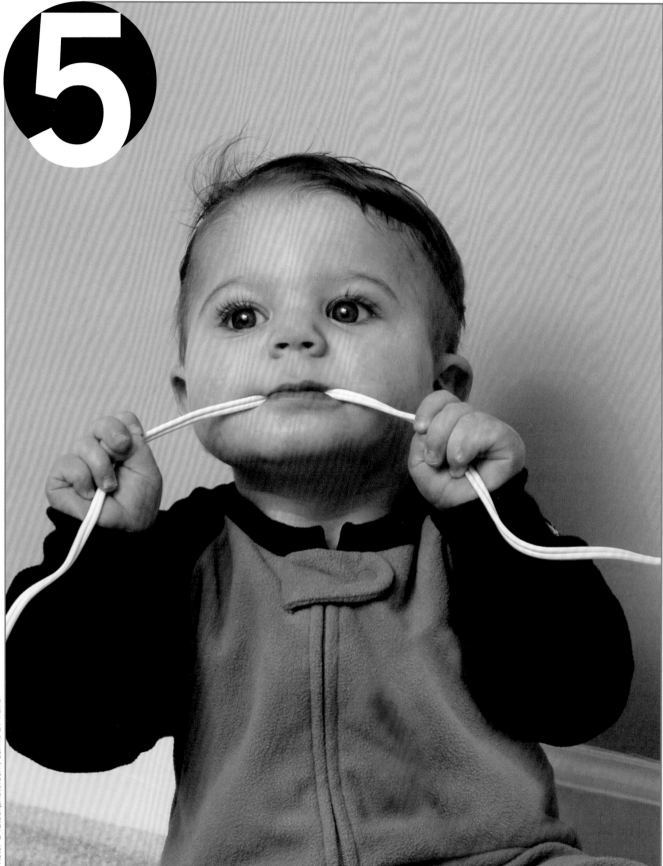

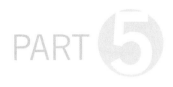

PART **5** # Safety at home and on the move

PART 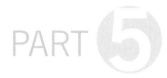 # Avoidable accidents

Introduction

Most car crashes happen within 100 yards of the home. With children under five, most accidents happen in the home. Like the automobile variety they occur very quickly and are more likely when adults are under stress, in a rush or when their usual routine is changed. Because you know your own home, you are in the best position to look out for possible dangers.

The kinds of accidents children have are related to their age or developmental stage so there are particular things to watch out for depending on the age of your child. Accidents range from the trivial bruise to the life-threatening burn. If a child can be distracted easily from their distress it is unlikely to be serious but never underestimate the stoicism of children, particularly when they may be feeling guilty over the accident. It can be very difficult to tell the difference between child abuse and an accident. Other children, including siblings, can be merciless and bite marks on babies from jealous brothers or sisters are not uncommon. Don't be surprised if the doctor or nurse asks you some searching questions should you turn up at casualty. Most departments have automatic referral systems to the social services for any fracture or serious injury to children. This can be very distressing for parents and for the social workers concerned.

Babies 0-1 year old

At this stage babies are able to wriggle, grasp, suck and roll over. There are a number of possible accidents that are common in this age group.

Suffocation and choking in babies

Babies can swallow, inhale or choke on items such as small toys, peanuts and marbles. Choose toys appropriate to the age of your baby. Look for: 'contains small parts unsuitable for small children' labels. Ensure that small objects such as marbles, peanuts and small toys are kept out of reach. Encourage older children to keep their toys away from your baby. Avoid pillows and soft bedding, don't put infants to sleep unattended in an adult bed or on the sofa.

Falls

Particularly likely if you leave your baby on a raised surface. Be sure, when you are changing nappies, that you avoid the baby rolling off a bed or sofa. You can use a baby mat on the floor. This also goes for the changing rooms in supermarkets and restraints.

Burns and scalds

Possible if your baby is near hot objects. Avoid hot or warm objects such as ovens, light bulbs, radiators, curling tongs, hairdryers, irons and fires. Place hot drinks out of your baby's reach. Fit short power leads on kettles and heaters. **Remember** hot water can scald up to 30 minutes after it has boiled.

Poisoning

Babies' natural instincts are to suck anything which comes into contact with their mouths. Many ordinary household substances can be poisonous, even iron tablets or salt.

All poisonous substances should be kept outside your baby's reach at all times. This includes medicines such as sleeping tablets which tend to be left on the bedroom table conveniently next to the bed.

Care should also be taken when washing babies' bottles, so that they do not come into contact with poisonous substances. Young brothers or sisters should be supervised when around babies to stop them feeding tablets or other poisonous substances to baby just to see what happens.

Children 1-4 years old

Once the mainframe computer kicks in with better acceleration toddlers can move very quickly, so accidents often happen in seconds. Unfortunately coordination comes later. As children get older they will explore more which means they are more likely to have knocks and bruises, not least from their adoring brothers and sisters. Keeping an eye on the wandering toddler and thinking ahead can be difficult but life-saving. Thankfully not that many kids turn up in casualty with pots stuck on their heads.

Falls

Although small children can squeeze their bodies through a gap as small as 100mm wide (smaller than the length of a teaspoon) they tend to get their heads trapped.

Check the width between railings, banisters and balconies and board them up if necessary. Fit window locks or safety catches that stop windows opening wider than 100mm.

Move furniture such as beds, sofas and chairs away from windows to prevent children climbing up and falling out.

Fit a safety gate at the bottom and top of the stairs, use a safety gate to keep small children out of the kitchen too. Make sure older children know they should keep the gate locked.

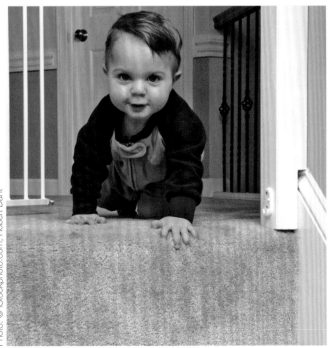

Keep stair gates shut

Burns and scalds

Any burn greater than the size of the child's hand needs the attention of a doctor. Unfortunately we do underestimate the danger from simple things like a cup of tea to a little body with such a small surface area.

Make sure that you use an appropriate fire guard for all fires. Fit a smoke alarm on each floor of your home and make sure you check that it is working properly on a weekly basis. It is a good idea to have a fire escape plan worked out and to tell your children what to do in case of a fire.

Place hot drinks out of children's reach. Fit short power leads on kettles and heaters. Use the rear hobs of the cooker, keeping pan handles turned away from the edge. Children are curious and will reach for handles of pans on the stove.

Poisoning

By the age of 18 months or earlier children can open containers and by 3 years they may also be able to open child resistant tops and child cupboard safety catches with impunity - next stop the Rubik's cube.

Keep household chemicals, medicines, alcohol and even cosmetics out of children's reach, preferably in a locked cupboard, lockable suitcase or cosmetics case.

Keep poisonous items out of children's reach

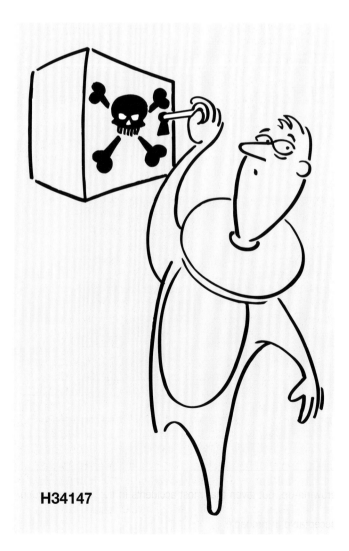

H34147

PART 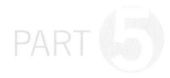 # Child protection at home

Introduction

Protecting our children from harm means more than just vaccinations. Every year one child in five has an accident at home which is serious enough to need the doctor or treatment in hospital. Most homes just aren't designed with the safety of toddlers as a first priority; the comfort and convenience of adults is the overriding factor. This can be seen when a house is up for sale. All the safety features which protect children are removed from sight just in case they should detract from the appearance of the house. Many people will take child guards away when they are expecting guests.

Designs for such things as stairs can take little regard of the probability that at some time there will be children in the house. Equally, people will accept designs for buildings to live in which ignore children because they either have none of their own or they have all grown up. Yet almost all houses will have children in them at some time; relatives, guests and visitors may all bring along their children. It is best to include the potential for such safety devices, even if they are not required immediately.

It's from the first day baby crawls (at about 9 months) up to the time a toddler learns to recognise some of the main dangers around him (at about 4 years) that your child is most at risk from an accident at home. Now that infectious diseases no longer pose such a threat (they were once the commonest cause of death for children under two years old), accidents present the greatest risk. Thankfully the loss of life and illness is not on the same scale but as most accidents are preventable, they represent a tragic game of chance for small children.

Natural curiosity, an innocent lack of fear, together with the unsteady process of learning to walk, all conspire to put toddlers at risk of injury from very ordinary, everyday things. Kettles, cups of tea, bath-water, heaters, stairs, windows, kitchen gadgets, cooking utensils, household DIY and garden chemicals, as well as the obvious hazards of medicines and drugs, all hold dangers for them.

Parents can do a great deal to reduce the risks faced by their children simply by being aware of where danger lurks. One way is to take a look round the house, room by room, to identify risks.

Many dangers can be removed at no expense. It may mean that adults have to put up with a less attractive or convenient home for a few years. But for the sake of a young child's safety and well-being surely that's a worthwhile sacrifice. Your child needs the freedom to explore your home in safety. Few would deny that bruises and sticking plaster are a natural part of growing-up, but given that most accidents in the home or garden can be prevented, serious injuries to children should be neither acceptable or probable.

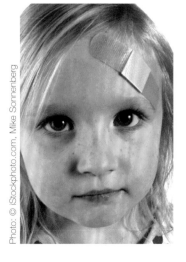

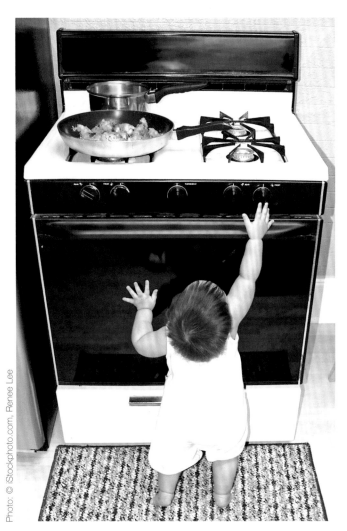

Cooker guards

Some of the most horrendous injuries to children occur in the kitchen or where there is unguarded equipment. Men are already aware of the danger but as we are spending increasingly more time in the kitchen, the dangers become more immediately obvious. There is now a wide range of protective guards and equipment designed to prevent burns and scalds caused by toddlers pulling hot utensils or kitchen gadgets and their contents over them. Three-quarters of serious scalds to one to four year olds involve spillage from cups, teapots, kettles and saucepans. A minor scald to an adult from a cup of tea can be lethal to a small baby because of their small surface area of skin.

Hob and cooker guards are normally easy to fit, but fitting a hob guard to a sealed hob can be more difficult. Remember though that the guard itself, along with the sides and doors of some cookers, can get very hot. Don't get lulled into a false sense of security. After fitting a cooker or hob guard, still take care to turn pan handles away from the edge.

Electricity

Long electric flexes which overhang work tops are particularly dangerous. They can be replaced with coiled cables which will retract after stretching. When contracted they are usually about 300mm, extending to 1 metre when stretched out. Some appliances will be made safer from their use, such as: electric kettles, coffee percolators, toasters and any other small appliances, especially those where existing flex hangs over work tops to attract inquisitive fingers. However, they are not an unmixed blessing. They have the annoying and potentially dangerous habit of entangling with other flexes, particularly others of the coiled variety. It is often best not to have two coiled flexes on the same double point as there is a temptation, as happens with the telephone, not to untangle the flex until it becomes too difficult to use. Also, the very appearance of these flexes is attractive to children who are used to toys in similar designs. As an alternative, consider cordless irons and kettles. They are a good investment despite their slightly higher price.

Houses are increasingly being fitted with residual current device (RCD) circuit breakers, also known as earth leakage trips. These units will detect extremely small currents leaking to earth and break the circuit almost instantly. If a child succeeds in circumventing all your best efforts at preventing electric shock, provided there is a good earth in the house and the equipment is correctly wired, they will not be killed by the shock. Even so, there is still a contact with the electric mains even though it is only for a fraction of a second. They will receive an electric shock which could cause them to fall or drop the apparatus, thus causing injury. Preventing a shock in the first place is still the name of the game.

Safety gates and barriers

Expecting children, particularly very young children, to use their common-sense with regard to dangerous areas, is forgetting the lemming-like regard such junior members of the human race have for personal safety. Gates or barriers should be used at the threshold of any danger for an unsteady toddler or a crawling baby. They are a must to prevent a baby falling down the stairs. You may also save injuries and worry if you put them in the doorway of the kitchen, the bathroom, at the back door and the doorway to the garage or tool-shed.

Make sure that the gate or barrier you buy is approved for the use to which it will be put, but remember that no BS number will protect your child from incorrect fitting. At the top of the stairs, gates which give way when pushed are potentially more dangerous than no gate at all. Similarly, having to climb over a gate which is too difficult to open presents a danger not only to an adult but also to the child they may be carrying in their arms. Older children will usually take the easiest route and simply clamber over the gate (or swing on it). If it is right on the edge of the flight of stairs, they too can easily fall.

A gate is a permanent fixture; it needs to be screwed into the wall, banisters or door posts, which in turn need to be stout enough to take the load. But it can be opened and closed easily and quickly to allow adults and older children through. Most gates swing both ways and can be hinged either side. One model folds up concertina fashion against the wall to allow adults to get through. Avoid self-closing varieties which may well close but fail to lock. They can also close with enough force to knock a small child backwards down the stairs.

When is a gate not a gate? When it is ajar, obviously. A gate is no use at all if you forget to close it properly. Training the older children into the habit of always closing doors along with gates will help keep the younger members of the family safe.

A barrier can be moved from place to place round the home but it must be carefully tightened up every time. Nevertheless, once firmly in place, you can be sure a toddler can't get through. Both barriers and gates come in a choice of wood or metal designs. Most barriers are simple to fix. They rely on rubber buffer tension fixing, so there is no need to screw anything into the walls or posts at each end. You may find barriers with only one buffer (rather than two) at each end more convenient.

Guards for heaters and fires

Children, like all animals, are fascinated by fire. For the stone-age father, it must have been a constant worry that Ug junior was about to fall into the flames. Sadly, injuries from fires still account for a very large proportion of childhood hospital visits. Strong, well-attached guards should be used anywhere there is a gas or electric heater, an open fire, wood or oil burning stove. Avoid the flimsy free-standing guards which are designed for appearance rather than their ability to protect. Look for a big all-round guard to protect toddlers both from the fire itself and from the hot casing or surround. Do not rely on the metal bars attached to the heater to protect your toddler; they can get very hot.

Open fires need the extra protection of a spark guard inside the main fire guard, but beware, spark guards themselves can get very hot. Bathing your baby in front of the fire is very pleasant but this too requires the use of a spark guard and a reasonable distance between the bath and the fire.

Portable heaters are particularly dangerous, so make sure they are well inside a guard which is fixed to the wall. For mobile gas cylinder heaters, use one of the guards designed specifically for them. Ideally, no part of the guard should be closer than 200mm from the heat source. Too close and the guard itself could get dangerously hot.

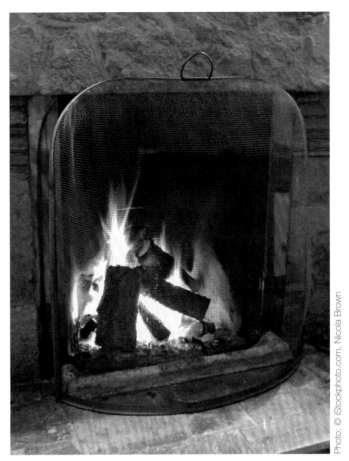

Many fire guards will still get hot

Photo: © iStockphoto.com, Nicola Brown

Window locks

Many landings in older houses have windows at floor or near floor level. It makes sense to protect these windows from children while at the same time allowing their use for ventilation and as fire escapes. Locks are better, therefore, than vertical bars because so long as you keep the key handy, the window can still provide an escape route if there's a fire.

If you don't like the idea of no fresh air in the room, consider those locks which can also set the window in a slightly open position. (The maximum safe opening for children is about 100mm) Even windows apparently out of reach can be a danger to children if there is furniture under windows for children to climb on to.

Having fire-practice drills can be great fun for the children. It establishes a pattern for them should there be a fire. It also helps identify those windows which will not open any more, usually after the last round of house painting.

Safety glass and film

Building regulations now dictate that all new houses, or glass replacement where children can reach, must be of a minimum thickness to prevent children from falling through the glass. It is difficult to overemphasise just how serious injury to children can

be from such an accident. Unfortunately, even the thicker glass is not unbreakable and the glass will leave pointed fragments within the frame. Safety glass is not only stronger than ordinary glass, but when it does break up it is much less likely to cause serious injury. Choose between laminated glass and toughened (tempered) safety glass.

Laminated glass is made from two sheets of ordinary glass with a sheet of plastic sandwiched and bonded between them. When it is damaged it stays in one piece, the glass being held together by the plastic inside. It can be cut and trimmed to size but not as easily as ordinary glass.

Safety film is a clear plastic film which is spread on to one surface of the existing glass in your home. It holds the glass together if it gets broken. Safety film is difficult to remove once properly in place. Safety film is cheaper than safety glass, but is less effective, particularly if incorrectly fitted. Both methods of protection are also useful as burglar deterrents but have the serious disadvantage of making escape from fire difficult if the window needs to be broken.

Medicines and dangerous chemicals

Every year a considerable number of children will eat, drink or pour medicine and chemicals over themselves. Children are naturally curious. It's a healthy instinct but unless you take precautions to keep dangerous things beyond their reach, there could be distinctly unhealthy results. Poisoning is one of the most common accidents amongst children between one and four years old.

The treatment necessary to save poison victims can be very frightening for toddlers. Washing out the stomach by passing a tube down their throat is standard for the non-toxic chemicals. Similarly, an emetic (a substance which makes them vomit) is often employed while they are fully conscious. For most forms of poisoning, blood samples will need to be taken. So it make sense to keep all drugs, pills and medicines, as well as household and garden chemicals, in child-resistant containers or firmly behind closed cupboard doors which children cannot open. Child resistant catches are cheap and easy to fit. It may be safer to keep garden and DIY chemicals under lock and key in the garden shed or garage.

Because medicines and drugs hold particular dangers for toddlers (pills look like sweets, medicines look like juice) you may want to keep all medicines, etc, in a lockable cabinet as a first priority.

One of the commonest causes of poisoning involves keeping dangerous chemicals such as weed-killers in lemonade bottles. You should never transfer chemicals from the bottles or packets they are sold in.

House fires

About 80 children die in house fires every year. This is the commonest cause of accidental death in the home for children. Your local fire station will help you with advice on fire prevention and planning fire escape. Your first priority if a fire occurs is to get everyone out as quickly as possible and not to try to put the fire out yourself. Once out of the house children should be kept somewhere safe and no attempt made to return inside the house. Many families have lost their father for the sake of a favourite toy or TV set.

A well-placed smoke detector alarm on every floor will wake you in the event of a fire. It will only do this, however, if it has power to work it. You should pick one day per week to check the batteries, turning it into a game for the children helps spread the load. Better still, install units which permanently charge from the mains. Even so, they will still need to be checked on a regular basis.

Sitting and playing

It seems incredible that many accidents and injury to babies occur during 'play-time'. It is often not the type of play which is the danger but rather the lack of supervision or the equipment being used in an inappropriate manner. Some play equipment has been found to be dangerous and is no longer recommended. This is particularly true of the baby walker – many of these items can, however, still be bought, particularly second-hand, and may even carry a BS number.

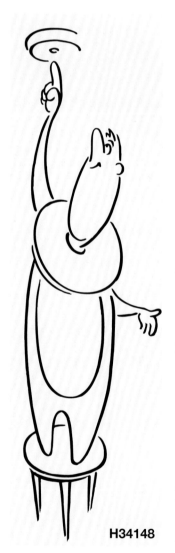

H34148

Check the smoke alarm batteries every week

PART 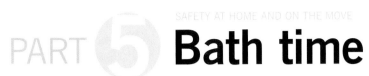 Bath time

At first you can bathe your baby in a hand basin, but you will find a purpose-made baby bath useful as the baby gets bigger. These baths are designed to minimise the amount of water used and keep the baby in an upright position. Obviously this will only be of value if you support a small baby while in the bath. Babies are unable to support themselves or lift themselves out of water so only a few centimetres of water are sufficient for drowning.

Baby baths are almost invariably made of plastic; this makes them very light when empty but they can also be very slippery. Despite the fact they will hold only a small amount of water, when full they can still be heavy to carry. Worse still, a bath with water plus baby is not only heavy but also slippery. It is always best to set the bath up in the position in which you wish to use it rather than carrying water and baby in it to a warm spot.

Many designs of bath are available. Some fit on the main bath, some have a separate stand and others form part of a changing unit. Whichever type you use, the closer it is to the floor, the better. Holding a baby covered in soap is like trying to hold on to ten eggs covered in oil. (You shouldn't be using soap on new-borns anyway.)

Check that the stand for the bath is solid and fits the bath well. This is particularly important if it is second-hand as the various connections may have become loose. If the bath is part of a changing unit, make sure the mat or cover lifts off or slides away completely, and cannot drop down onto your baby while he is in the bath.

Never leave a child unattended in the bath even for a moment.

Always add the hot water to cold water in the bath. Even a small amount of hot water can cause a severe scald in a child as they have such a small surface area of skin. Use a non-slip bath liner to help prevent your baby from slipping.

A wet baby covered in soap bubbles, sat in the bath in front of the fire, makes an attractive sight. It is worth remembering, however, just how dangerous fires of all kinds can be to a small child. Sparks from an open fire, or even worse, the baby able to reach the fire, are very real dangers. Electric fires or fan heaters have no place near water, which your baby will make sure is spread liberally about the room.

Keep the bath away from hazards which your baby might reach by standing in the bath or climbing onto the edge of it. Keep the bath away from the taps, not only to prevent them from being turning on but also to stop the hot tap being touched - it may remain very hot some time after use.

Once your child starts to pull himself up, stop using the baby bath on a stand or in the sink. Either use an adult bath or put the baby bath inside the adult bath. Adult baths are perfectly safe if all the precautions are observed for bathing the baby in any form of bath. However, they can be made from steel or cast iron and can be dangerous to fall onto. Lifting a slippery baby out needs just that bit more care.

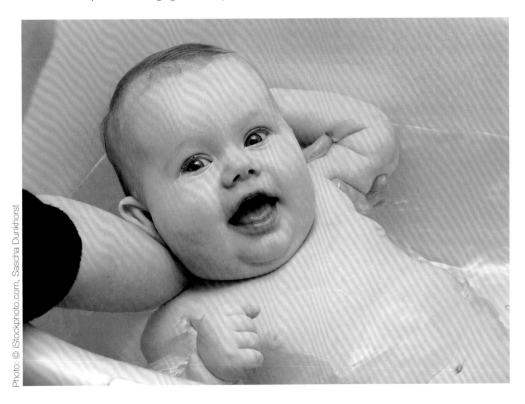

Photo: © iStockphoto.com, Sascha Dunkhorst

PART 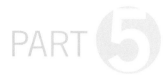 # Moses baskets and cribs

Introduction

Newborn babies are going to be moved around quite a bit, not least to keep a close watch on them at all times no matter where you are. Although neither item is an essential buy, Moses baskets and cribs can make life easier as they are designed for use during your baby's first few months by providing a small cosy and portable environment for a newborn.

> Always, always buy a new mattress for the cot. No exceptions. Same for the crib.

It is tempting to buy some of this equipment second-hand, and indeed it makes good economic sense. However, don't buy a second-hand mattress - older ones may not conform to the latest safety and toxicity standards.

Moses baskets

These are very portable and fit easily into your own bedroom, the ideal place for early days. Moses baskets come in a variety of styles.

Check out:
- Is the mattress included?
- Is a stand included?
- Is a linen set included?
- Is there an optional hood or any features?
- Are the handles strong enough for repeated carrying?
- Is it fire resistant?

Note
Don't place on the floor – use a stand.

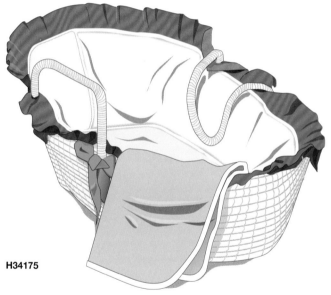

H34175

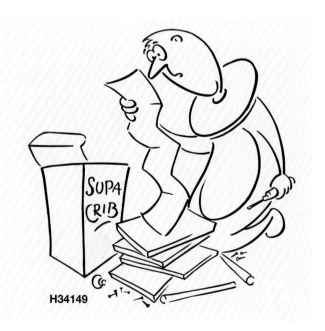

H34149

Cribs

The bad news about cribs is that they often come as flat-pack pieces of furniture which have to be assembled. Watch out for the inevitable three screws and a split pin left over. Cribs are suitable for a baby up to around six months and should not be used once they can sit up, kneel or attain an upright position on their own.

Check out:
- Does it come with a mattresses?
- Are there drape rails to attach drapes to create a hood above the head end of the crib?
- You will almost always need to buy bedding separately.

PART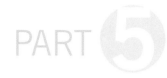

Baby bouncers

Anything which gives bouncing movement is bound to be a hit with babies. This is even better if they can add their own movement despite their relatively weak legs. For very young babies there are swings that can be used inside. Gone are the days when you simply fastened a glorified seat to the door frame with elastic, they now come with automatic timing mechanisms, multi-speed options, padded reclining seats, added activity features, and are allegedly suitable from birth. Be aware though that not all experts endorse their use, on the grounds that they can put weight on the baby's legs, and associated stress on the leg muscles, at an earlier age than would happen naturally through learning to walk.

For older babies you can use more robust traditional swings or bouncers. These are hung from a door frame and allow the child to feel their feet and begin to get the idea for walking while being fully and safely supported.

Caution: The door frames in modern houses may not be capable of taking the load of a baby bouncer. Get expert advice, or use a free-standing type.

There is a huge amount of choice but make safety the number one priority and look for:
● Safe, securing mechanisms.
● Supportive, comfy seats.
● Correct amount of bounce for the age of the baby.

Note
After many accidents, baby walkers are now considered too unsafe by most professionals. They may also delay walking.

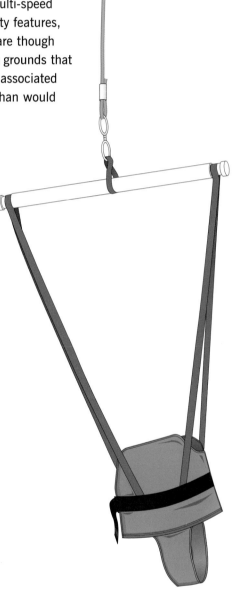

H34178

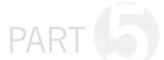 PART

High chairs

Despite all the revolutions in baby care there are some things which remain more or less the same for decades. High chairs create a safe, hygienic environment where babies can eat. They are also very good for your back. Most importantly they allow the baby to be at eye level with the rest of the family. There will be a time when they will refuse to use one and will make it very clear that they wish to sit with everyone else.

High chairs allow the baby to be at the same level as the rest of the family

A plastic seat which straps onto a normal chair is handy, especially when visiting people who don't have children (although tempting, only put the child in it for snacks/drinks/meals as they become rather loud if strapped in for long periods!).

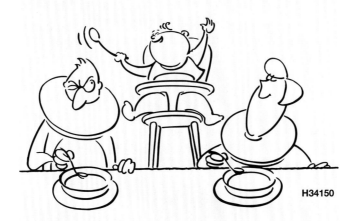

H34150

There is a great deal of choice but watch out for:
- How big is it? Can you store/transport it easily?
- Can you remove the seat cover to clean it?
- Does it recline?
- Can you fasten the baby in for safety?

High chair which converts to chair and table

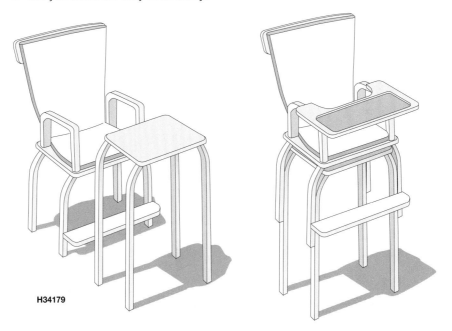

H34179

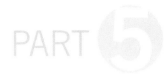

PART **5**

Playpens

You may find a playpen a useful place for your baby to play near you, but away from dangers. Some playpens have wooden bars. Others have soft sides made out of mesh fabric. Make sure the playpen is at least 600mm deep, otherwise your child could climb over the edge and fall. This is particularly important because most injuries with playpens occur when the child climbs out or gets stuck in the bars of the pen.

Safety first
● Keep the mesh sides up all the time. If the side is down, a child inside the playpen could crawl into the pocket made by the fabric side and suffocate. A child outside the playpen could trap a hand in the folding mechanism.
● Always watch your child if there are large toys or boxes in the playpen. They could be used as steps to climb out.
● If you tie toys to the playpen, only use strings shorter than 300mm. Longer strings can strangle.
● Don't tie toys across the top of the playpen.

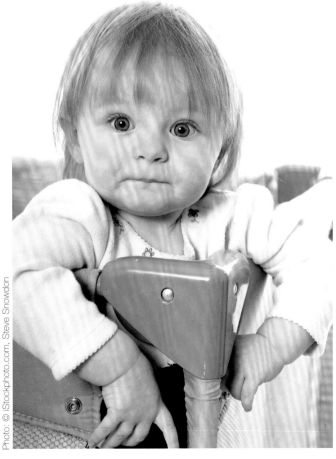

Photo: © iStockphoto.com, Steve Snowdon

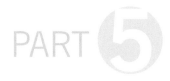

PART **5**

Getting from A to B with baby intact

Introduction

Once upon a time you carried a baby or toddler in your arms while in the car, not least because there was no choice. Unfortunately we learn the hard way and now there are specialised safety systems to protect your child. Similarly, babies were left to wander around homes with stairs mountaineers would look twice at.

Buggies

These devices grew out of a need for lighter more versatile transport than the pram. They are generally a lightweight, quick to fold, push-and-go-anywhere vehicle designed as much for ease of use as storage. They can collapse into a long-thin shape (umbrella folding), or may fold flat. Frankly, there is little other option for a dad who is going to use public transport or travel overseas. Airlines generally welcome them but only in the hold. Car use is also made easier, especially when compared with trying to get a rigid pushchair into the boot, unless you own a very large 4x4.

The buggy is an evolution of the pram

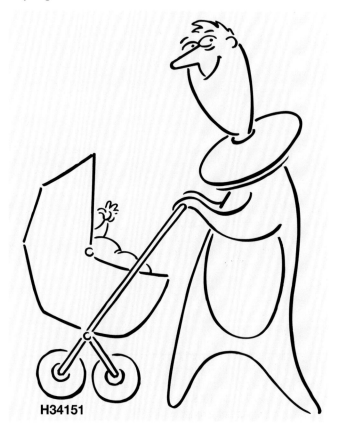

H34151

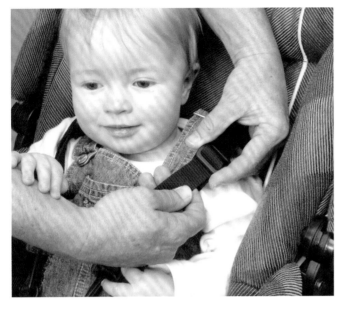

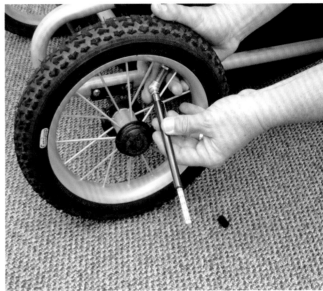

Ease of harness adjustment is important

There is a huge variety of options for buggies. Look out for:
● Buggies which fully recline as they are suitable from birth. The most basic models do not recline and are only suitable from age three to six months.
● Ease of opening and collapse.
● Lightweight.
● Freestanding and stable when collapsed. (Some will infuriatingly run away on two wheels.)
● Washable covers.
● Five-point harness, easily adjusted.
● Guarantee.
● On/off swivel on the front wheels. Vital for supermarkets/long walks.
● Blow-up tyres give a more comfortable ride than solid ones. They also make for easier pushing, but only if you keep them blown up.

Keep the tyres blown up for a comfortable ride and reduced pushing effort

Double pushchairs

If you need one of these, congratulations, you have just entered the equivalent of the two car family. There are variations on the theme of getting two children into essentially one machine:
● Facing each other.
● In-line with both facing front/rear.
● Side-by-side with two pushchairs joined together.
● Side-by-side with one very wide pushchair for two.

Twins will grow at the same rate, so the side-by-side options or in-line work equally well. Children of different ages can be more tricky and tend to need more cumbersome machines, but generally side-by-side models may be too wide to fit through shop doors. Face to face, in-line models are narrower and therefore easier to take into shops, but they may be quickly outgrown if there's not enough leg room.

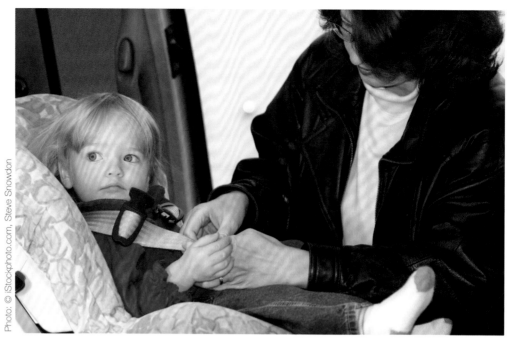

Photo: © iStockphoto.com, Steve Snowdon

Car seats

Car seats must always be used and be certified to the latest European standard (UN ECE R44.03) or better, although a child is still far safer in any car seat than in no car seat at all. Beware second-hand car seats though unless you are perfectly sure of their history - for instance if they are from another family member.

There are some exceptions to using a car seat: in the rear of a taxi or in an emergency vehicle.

Some things are more than simply desirable:

● The seat must be the correct size for your child.
● The seat must surround the child's head.
● The seat must fit into your car correctly and into any other car you are likely to use it in. It is worth asking the retailer to demonstrate how the seat fits and to check that it is suitable for your vehicle(s).
● Securing clamps must stay in place if the seat is to stay safe. Get advice from a qualified mechanic if necessary.
● The shoulder harness must allow for growth by maintaining a correct fit over the shoulders.
● Padded harnesses prevent chest damage on impact.
● Unless impossible to fit you should always favour rearward-facing seats, which generally offer better protection than forward-facing models, particularly in front impact accidents.
● Never use a child seat in the front of a car equipped with airbags, unless the passenger airbag can be disabled. See your car's handbook, or your Haynes car manual, for details.

Baby carriers

Even more than pushing a pram, a man would never have been seen dead with one of these devices for carrying a small baby. Times change, and so does your choice.

Their big plus is versatility – you can wander around with the baby on your back or front with no need for a buggy. The ultimate off-road system where you supply the torque and traction. They can carry a baby from birth and many newborn

Using a typical baby carrier. Always refer to the manufacturer's instructions for details specific to your model

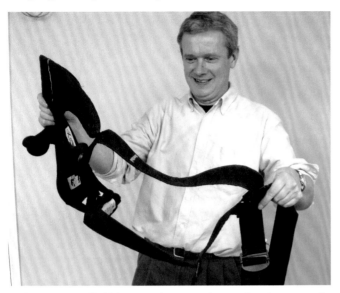

1   Remind yourself which way up it goes; make sure the straps are not twisted

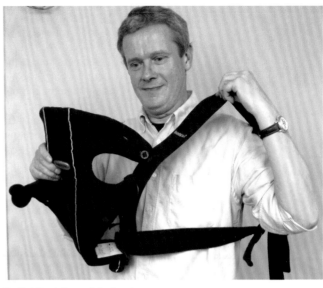

2   Put the left arm into the straps . . .

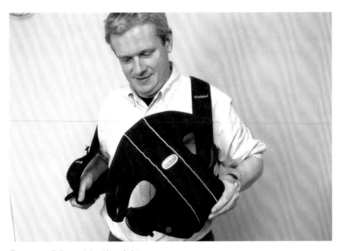

3   . . . followed by the right arm . . .

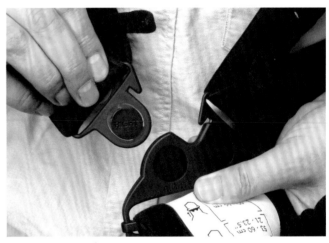

4   . . . and secure the buckle

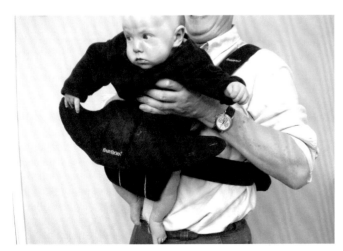

5   Insert the baby . . .

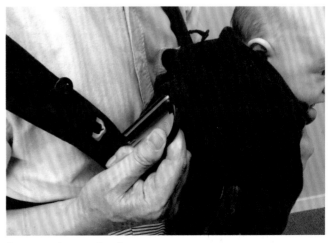

6   . . . and secure the sling

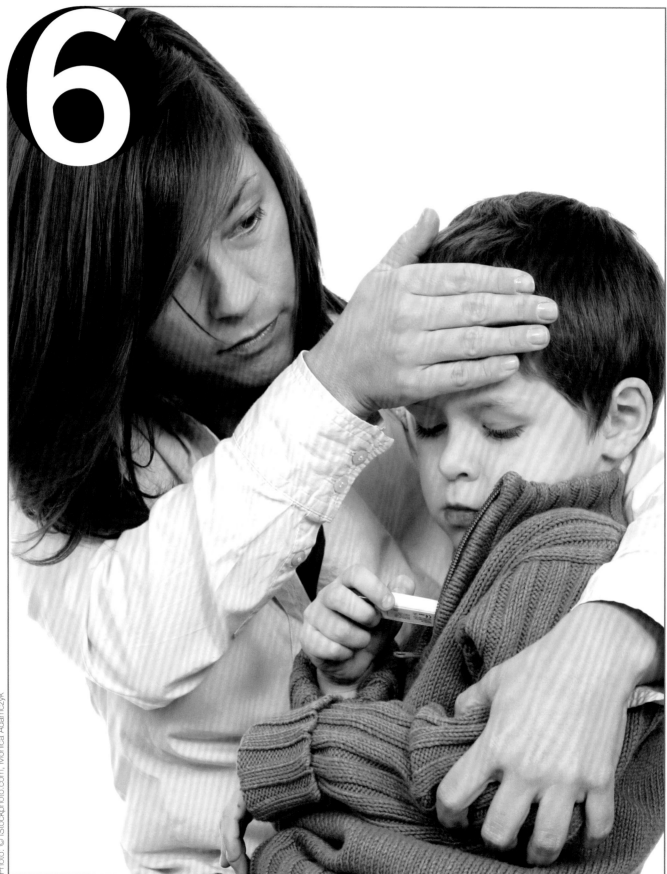

6

PART 6 Childhood ailments

PART 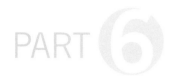 # General

Introduction

Most accidental injuries are minor and can be treated using simple first aid measures, but in the unlikely event of a serious accident or sudden illness, knowledge of first aid techniques could help you to save your child's life. You should get professional training rather than waiting for it to happen first.

By following the basic guidelines provided here you will be able to deal with most day-to-day accidents and injuries. Information on dealing with emergencies is also provided.

To get more detailed information, and training in emergency first aid, contact the British Red Cross or St John Ambulance (see *Contacts* on page 193).

The key things to remember in any emergency situation are:
● Remain calm and confident.
● Do all you can to help but don't put yourself in danger.
● Do not give the injured person anything to eat or drink.

Emergencies

Seek **URGENT** medical attention for:
● Head injury with bleeding from eyes, ears or nose, drowsiness or vomiting.
● Loss of consciousness.
● Broken bone or dislocation.
● Severe chest pain or breathlessness.
● Sudden severe abdominal pain that won't go away.
● Unresolved choking and difficulty breathing.
● Severe bleeding.

Getting help

Sometimes, the quickest way of getting medical help is to take the child directly to the accident department of your local hospital. But call an ambulance and do not move the child if:
● You think they have a back or neck injury, or any other injury that could be made worse by movement.
● The child is unconscious or has stopped breathing, and needs your constant attention.

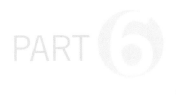

PART **6** # How to deal with an emergency

The recovery position

This is a safe position for an unconscious casualty, which allows easy breathing and prevents choking if they vomit. The details are different according to the age of the child, but the principle is the same.

Babies (up to 1 year old)

Place the baby face down on your forearm, with arms and legs dangling. Support the baby's head with your hand. Make sure that the child's tongue is not obstructing breathing.

Children (1 year and above)

After checking they are breathing normally, turn them on their side. Ensure that the airway is clear, with the jaw pulled forward and their head tipped slightly back.

Mouth-to-mouth resuscitation (kiss of life)

Note: *There is a risk of damaging a baby's lungs by blowing into the mouth. Better to let your chest fall naturally without forcing the breath out.*

Check first for anything obstructing the airway inside the mouth.
- Place the baby on a firm surface. Tilt back the head and lift the chin to open the air passages.
- Check for 10 seconds to see if they are breathing. If they are, place them in the recovery position described above.
- Cover the mouth and nose with your mouth (or just the nose if you cannot make a good seal) and give a gentle breath. Their chest should rise.
- Allow their chest to fall and give five more breaths (at about 20 per minute).
- Check whether they are breathing on their own. If not, continue.

Cardio-pulmonary resuscitation (CPR)

If there is still no breathing, start CPR. Remember it is different for babies and small children.
- Place the baby in the same position as for mouth-to-mouth resuscitation.
- Imagine a line between the baby's nipples. Place two fingertips just below the mid-point of this line.
- Press at the rate of 100 per minute (in time with 'Nelly the Elephant'), moving the chest down no more than 20mm with each press.
- Give 30 compressions to 2 mouth-to-mouth breaths.
    For small children proceed as above, but use one hand instead of two fingertips and move the chest downwards no more than 30mm.
    While you are doing this, someone else should be telephoning 999/112 for an ambulance. Keep other important numbers readily available.

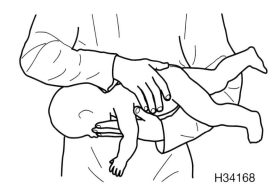
H34168

Recovery position for babies

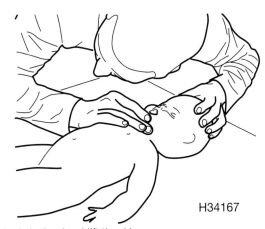
H34167

Tilt back the head and lift the chin to open the air passages

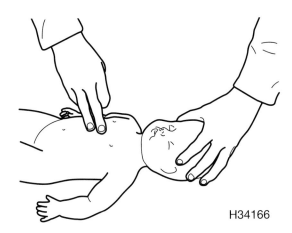
H34166

CPR point for babies. Only use two fingers, not the whole hand

PART 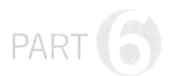 # Is your baby really ill?

Parents are usually good at noticing when something is wrong with their baby, but it is common not to be sure whether there is something really wrong.

Look out for these important signs and call your doctor or NHS Direct (0845 46 47).

Something wrong with the baby's response to you such as:

- When awake, your baby may seem unusually drowsy or not interested in looking at you.
- Not interested in feeding.
- When cuddled, your baby feels floppy or limp.
- Crying seems different (perhaps moaning, whimpering or shrill), and soothing doesn't help.

Other signs of illness

If you are already worried and then notice other problems too (like those in the list below), call your doctor or NHS Direct (0845 46 47) for advice.

- Is your baby very pale?
- Is your baby irritable and does not like being touched?
- Is there a new rash starting to appear?
- Is there bruised or discoloured look to the skin?
- Is there a fever?
- Is there difficulty with breathing or is breathing much faster than usual?
- Is your baby being sick (vomiting)?

A fever can be a sign that something is wrong. Anything over 38°C (100°F) is cause for concern

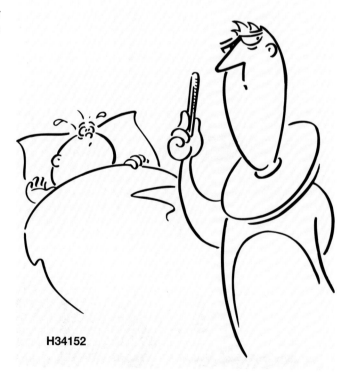

H34152

PART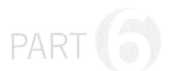

Taking a young child to hospital

If you and your child need to go to hospital:

● Reassure your child and explain that you're going together to see the doctor at the hospital to make things better.
● Take a favourite toy with you.
● Dress your child in a coat or a dressing gown over their nightclothes, or dress your child fully (it doesn't matter which, do what seems most sensible).
● Arrange care for other children or, if this is not possible, take them as well (it is not wise to leave a child at home without an adult there to look after them).

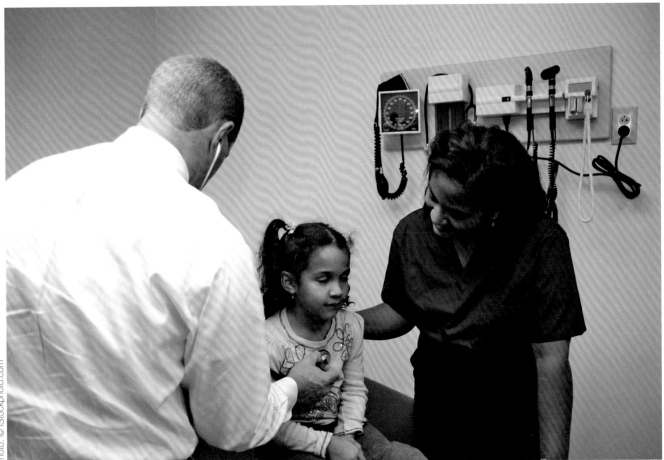

Photo: © iStockphoto.com

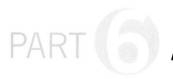

PART **6** # Antibiotics

Introduction

In the vast majority of cases, children will get better without antibiotics, so it makes sense for your doctor not to prescribe them. Their body's defence system can often protect against infection without the need for antibiotics which are being prescribed far too much.

Don't always expect to be given a prescription as doctors need to prescribe antibiotics with care, not least because inappropriate use of antibiotics can be dangerous for individual patients and for the whole population. Overuse of antibiotics can also cause resistance and result in them not working in the future. This is a very worrying trend, especially for patients with serious life-threatening infections.

Antibiotic facts

- Antibiotics have no effect on viral infections (eg colds, flu and most sore throats). Viral infections are much more common than bacterial infections.
- Inappropriate use of antibiotics can encourage the development of resistant bacteria. This could mean that the antibiotic may not work when your child really needs it.
- Some antibiotics have harmful side-effects such as diarrhoea and allergic reactions.
- Antibiotics do not just attack the infection they are prescribed for, they can also kill useful bacteria which protect against other infections such as thrush.

There are effective alternative remedies for managing the symptoms of many infections.

If your baby or child is prescribed antibiotics, ensure that they are given the medication according to instructions.

Although they may begin to feel better, they must take the full course of antibiotics to prevent their illness coming back.

Not taking the full course of antibiotics may lead to future antibiotic resistance.

If there is an infection such as a cold, flu or sore throat:
- Give paracetamol or paediatric ibuprofen according to the instructions to help reduce fever and relieve aches and pains.
- Give plenty of water to avoid dehydration.
- Ask your pharmacist (chemist) for advice. Many infections can be managed effectively with over-the-counter medications. The pharmacist will refer you to your doctor or practice nurse if they think it is necessary.

When to contact your GP

Call your GP's surgery for advice if, after taking over-the-counter medications as directed, your child is experiencing any of the following:
- Symptoms which are severe or unusually prolonged.
- Shortness of breath.
- Coughing up of blood or large amounts of yellow or green phlegm.

Harmful side-effects

Potential side-effects are another reason why doctors are cautious about prescribing antibiotics. Some antibiotic treatment can cause side-effects such as stomach upset and thrush. More serious side-effects which can be life-threatening can also happen.

PART **6** # Digestion problems

Gastroenteritis

Gastroenteritis simply means an inflammation of the stomach and the intestine which may cause vomiting and diarrhoea. Fortunately these attacks do tend to clear up on their own, but if the diarrhoea and vomiting are severe, dehydration can occur which can be serious, particularly in a baby.

Symptoms

Obviously a young baby cannot tell you about the pain that gastroenteritis can cause although they will tend to cry persistently. There is often a high temperature along with diarrhoea and vomiting, which can lead to serious dehydration if prolonged. If the baby still has open gaps in the skull bones (the soft areas of the scalp – fontanelles) these may be sunken when felt with your finger tip. In the older baby or child you may notice dark concentrated urine, a furred tongue and general malaise.

Causes

Viruses such as rotaviruses, commonly found in infected shellfish, are a common cause in the older child. Bacteria and other organisms can also cause gastroenteritis. These can be picked up from contaminated food or water and may reflect poor hygiene during food preparation. Not all cases of diarrhoea when away on holiday to another country are actually 'gastroenteritis'. The organisms which normally live in our bowels and do no harm are often replaced by the 'local' variety and diarrhoea can occur during this phase.

Failing to sterilise the baby's bottle correctly or making up the feed without taking care over hygiene can cause gastroenteritis. Contrary to popular myth, microwave ovens are not a good way of sterilising bottles unless used with a steriliser specifically designed for this method.

Diagnosis

Generally this is fairly obvious and is based on the symptoms, but any sign of dehydration in children must be acted on quickly (see *Fever* on page 182, *Diarrhoea* on page 151 and *Vomiting in children* on page 154).

Treatment and prevention

The name of the game is to replace lost fluids so diluting feeds, allowing more and longer breast feeds or giving rehydration mixtures as advised by your doctor helps replace lost fluid in young children and babies. If they are unable to take fluids for any reason such as repeated vomiting you should call your doctor. Do not give fizzy drinks, even after allowing them to go flat, as the sugar content can actually make the symptoms worse.

Anti-diarrhoeal medicine should not be given to babies. Some may be dangerous. Antibiotics are of no value in most cases of gastroenteritis, particularly those caused by viruses, and indeed can even make things worse.

Worms

Unfortunately common, particularly in young children, worms are not a sign of poor hygiene or bad living. Threadworms are the most common type of worm and cause itchy bottoms but are actually harmless. Roundworms are larger but less common. Tapeworms are much less common but can still be found in some parts of the UK.

Symptoms

Threadworms or roundworms can be seen in the baby's or child's motions as tiny white/brown worms in the stool. Night-time is the worst for itchiness as the female lays its eggs at the anus at this time causing the child to scratch, pick up the eggs, and pass them on or re-infect themselves.

Causes

Worms spread very quickly once within a family and can remain in families for considerable periods of time without anybody realising it. They usually infect children from contact with another child, who then passes it on to the other members of the family. Treating the whole family makes good sense therefore.

Prevention

- Wash your children's hands after using the potty or toilet as well as your own.
- Wash their and your hands before eating.
- Wash their and your hands after handling animals.

Treatment and self care

Use inverted adhesive tape (as you would for removing fluff from a jacket) to pick up worms or eggs from around the child's back passage. Bring it with you to your doctor who will prescribe medicine which works very effectively.

Abdominal pain

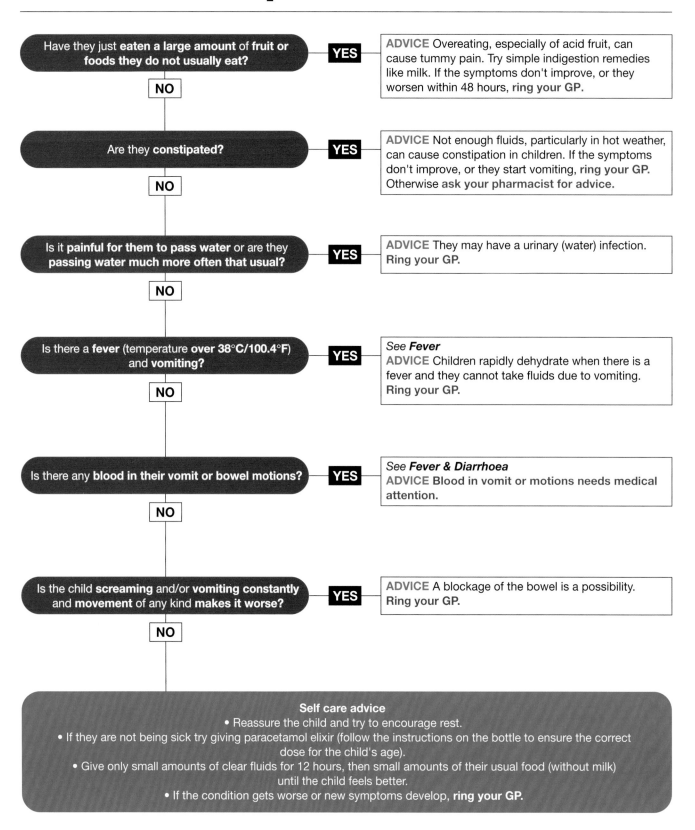

Have they just **eaten a large amount** of **fruit or foods they do not usually eat?**

YES → **ADVICE** Overeating, especially of acid fruit, can cause tummy pain. Try simple indigestion remedies like milk. If the symptoms don't improve, or they worsen within 48 hours, **ring your GP.**

NO ↓

Are they **constipated?**

YES → **ADVICE** Not enough fluids, particularly in hot weather, can cause constipation in children. If the symptoms don't improve, or they start vomiting, **ring your GP.** Otherwise **ask your pharmacist for advice.**

NO ↓

Is it **painful for them to pass water** or are they **passing water much more often that usual?**

YES → **ADVICE** They may have a urinary (water) infection. Ring your GP.

NO ↓

Is there a **fever** (temperature **over 38°C/100.4°F**) and **vomiting?**

YES → See **Fever**
ADVICE Children rapidly dehydrate when there is a fever and they cannot take fluids due to vomiting. Ring your GP.

NO ↓

Is there any **blood in their vomit or bowel motions?**

YES → See **Fever & Diarrhoea**
ADVICE Blood in vomit or motions needs medical attention.

NO ↓

Is the child **screaming** and/or **vomiting constantly** and **movement** of any kind **makes it worse?**

YES → **ADVICE** A blockage of the bowel is a possibility. Ring your GP.

NO ↓

Self care advice
• Reassure the child and try to encourage rest.
• If they are not being sick try giving paracetamol elixir (follow the instructions on the bottle to ensure the correct dose for the child's age).
• Give only small amounts of clear fluids for 12 hours, then small amounts of their usual food (without milk) until the child feels better.
• If the condition gets worse or new symptoms develop, **ring your GP.**

Diarrhoea

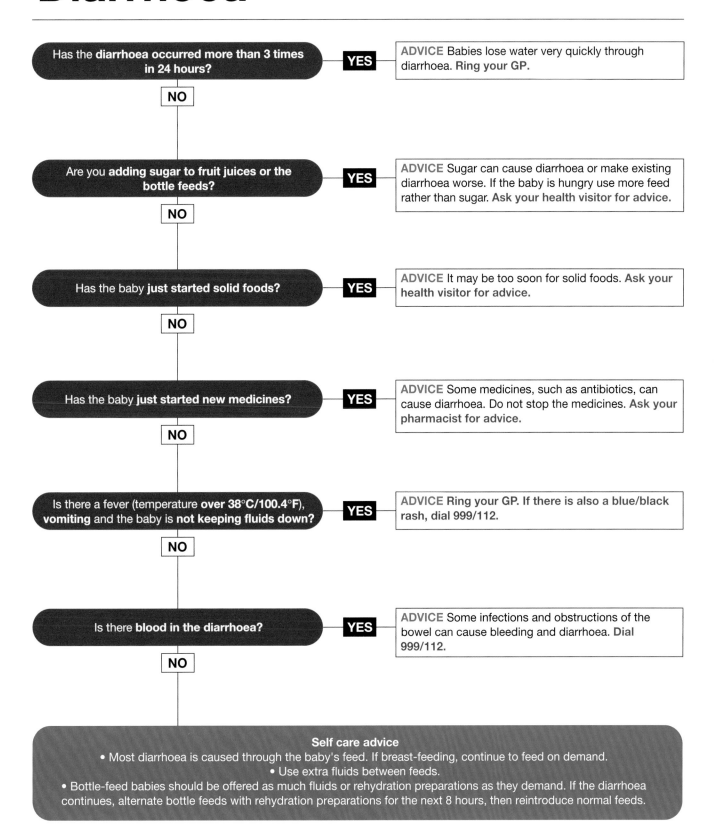

Has the diarrhoea occurred more than 3 times in 24 hours?

YES → **ADVICE** Babies lose water very quickly through diarrhoea. **Ring your GP.**

NO ↓

Are you adding sugar to fruit juices or the bottle feeds?

YES → **ADVICE** Sugar can cause diarrhoea or make existing diarrhoea worse. If the baby is hungry use more feed rather than sugar. **Ask your health visitor for advice.**

NO ↓

Has the baby just started solid foods?

YES → **ADVICE** It may be too soon for solid foods. **Ask your health visitor for advice.**

NO ↓

Has the baby just started new medicines?

YES → **ADVICE** Some medicines, such as antibiotics, can cause diarrhoea. Do not stop the medicines. **Ask your pharmacist for advice.**

NO ↓

Is there a fever (temperature over 38°C/100.4°F), vomiting and the baby is not keeping fluids down?

YES → **ADVICE** Ring your GP. If there is also a blue/black rash, dial 999/112.

NO ↓

Is there blood in the diarrhoea?

YES → **ADVICE** Some infections and obstructions of the bowel can cause bleeding and diarrhoea. **Dial 999/112.**

NO ↓

Self care advice
• Most diarrhoea is caused through the baby's feed. If breast-feeding, continue to feed on demand.
• Use extra fluids between feeds.
• Bottle-feed babies should be offered as much fluids or rehydration preparations as they demand. If the diarrhoea continues, alternate bottle feeds with rehydration preparations for the next 8 hours, then reintroduce normal feeds.

Poisoning

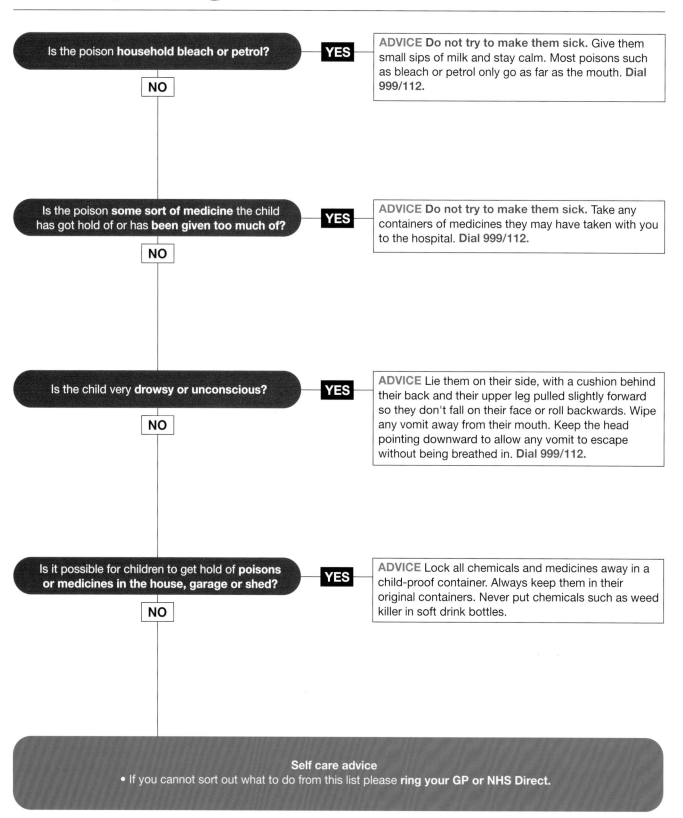

Is the poison **household bleach or petrol?** — **YES**

ADVICE Do not try to make them sick. Give them small sips of milk and stay calm. Most poisons such as bleach or petrol only go as far as the mouth. **Dial 999/112.**

NO

Is the poison **some sort of medicine** the child has got hold of or has **been given too much of?** — **YES**

ADVICE Do not try to make them sick. Take any containers of medicines they may have taken with you to the hospital. **Dial 999/112.**

NO

Is the child very **drowsy or unconscious?** — **YES**

ADVICE Lie them on their side, with a cushion behind their back and their upper leg pulled slightly forward so they don't fall on their face or roll backwards. Wipe any vomit away from their mouth. Keep the head pointing downward to allow any vomit to escape without being breathed in. **Dial 999/112.**

NO

Is it possible for children to get hold of **poisons or medicines in the house, garage or shed?** — **YES**

ADVICE Lock all chemicals and medicines away in a child-proof container. Always keep them in their original containers. Never put chemicals such as weed killer in soft drink bottles.

NO

Self care advice
• If you cannot sort out what to do from this list please **ring your GP or NHS Direct.**

Vomiting in babies

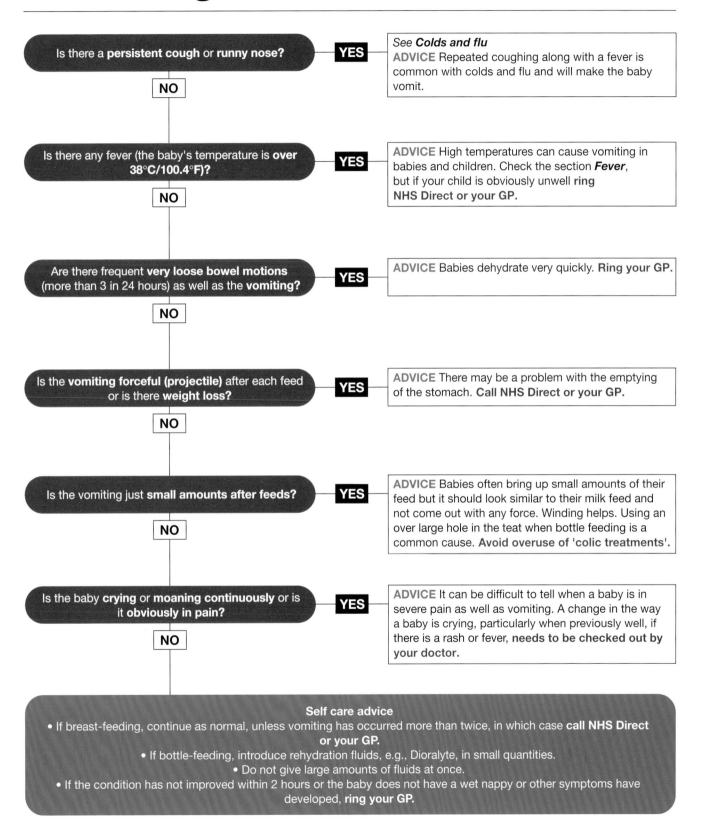

Is there a persistent cough or runny nose? — **YES**

> *See Colds and flu*
> **ADVICE** Repeated coughing along with a fever is common with colds and flu and will make the baby vomit.

NO

Is there any fever (the baby's temperature is over 38°C/100.4°F)? — **YES**

> **ADVICE** High temperatures can cause vomiting in babies and children. Check the section *Fever*, but if your child is obviously unwell **ring NHS Direct or your GP.**

NO

Are there frequent very loose bowel motions (more than 3 in 24 hours) as well as the vomiting? — **YES**

> **ADVICE** Babies dehydrate very quickly. **Ring your GP.**

NO

Is the vomiting forceful (projectile) after each feed or is there weight loss? — **YES**

> **ADVICE** There may be a problem with the emptying of the stomach. **Call NHS Direct or your GP.**

NO

Is the vomiting just small amounts after feeds? — **YES**

> **ADVICE** Babies often bring up small amounts of their feed but it should look similar to their milk feed and not come out with any force. Winding helps. Using an over large hole in the teat when bottle feeding is a common cause. **Avoid overuse of 'colic treatments'.**

NO

Is the baby crying or moaning continuously or is it obviously in pain? — **YES**

> **ADVICE** It can be difficult to tell when a baby is in severe pain as well as vomiting. A change in the way a baby is crying, particularly when previously well, if there is a rash or fever, **needs to be checked out by your doctor.**

NO

Self care advice
- If breast-feeding, continue as normal, unless vomiting has occurred more than twice, in which case **call NHS Direct or your GP.**
- If bottle-feeding, introduce rehydration fluids, e.g., Dioralyte, in small quantities.
- Do not give large amounts of fluids at once.
- If the condition has not improved within 2 hours or the baby does not have a wet nappy or other symptoms have developed, **ring your GP.**

Vomiting in children

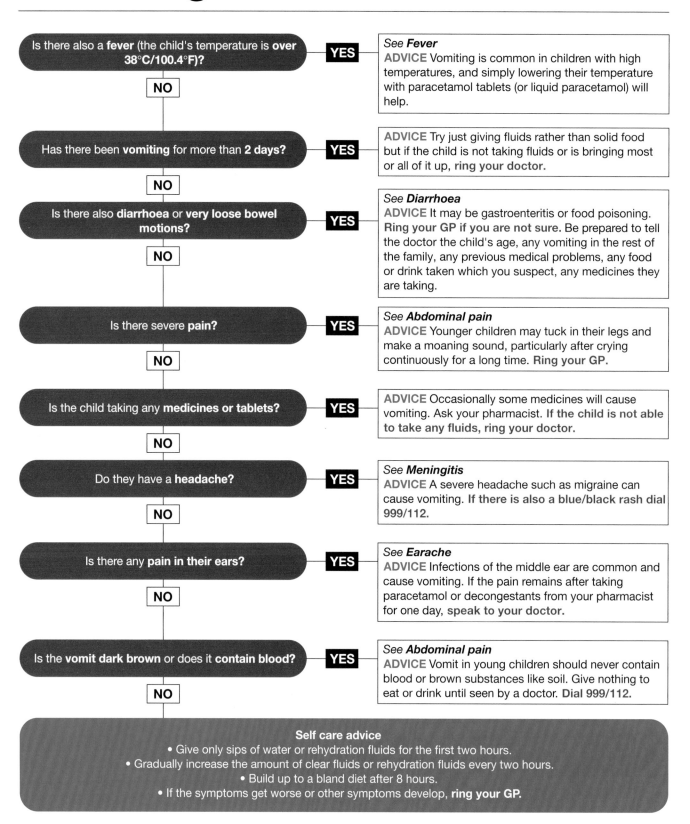

Is there also a fever (the child's temperature is over 38°C/100.4°F)? — **YES**

See Fever
ADVICE Vomiting is common in children with high temperatures, and simply lowering their temperature with paracetamol tablets (or liquid paracetamol) will help.

NO

Has there been vomiting for more than 2 days? — **YES**

ADVICE Try just giving fluids rather than solid food but if the child is not taking fluids or is bringing most or all of it up, **ring your doctor.**

NO

Is there also diarrhoea or very loose bowel motions? — **YES**

See Diarrhoea
ADVICE It may be gastroenteritis or food poisoning. **Ring your GP if you are not sure.** Be prepared to tell the doctor the child's age, any vomiting in the rest of the family, any previous medical problems, any food or drink taken which you suspect, any medicines they are taking.

NO

Is there severe pain? — **YES**

See Abdominal pain
ADVICE Younger children may tuck in their legs and make a moaning sound, particularly after crying continuously for a long time. **Ring your GP.**

NO

Is the child taking any medicines or tablets? — **YES**

ADVICE Occasionally some medicines will cause vomiting. Ask your pharmacist. **If the child is not able to take any fluids, ring your doctor.**

NO

Do they have a headache? — **YES**

See Meningitis
ADVICE A severe headache such as migraine can cause vomiting. **If there is also a blue/black rash dial 999/112.**

NO

Is there any pain in their ears? — **YES**

See Earache
ADVICE Infections of the middle ear are common and cause vomiting. If the pain remains after taking paracetamol or decongestants from your pharmacist for one day, **speak to your doctor.**

NO

Is the vomit dark brown or does it contain blood? — **YES**

See Abdominal pain
ADVICE Vomit in young children should never contain blood or brown substances like soil. Give nothing to eat or drink until seen by a doctor. **Dial 999/112.**

NO

Self care advice
- Give only sips of water or rehydration fluids for the first two hours.
- Gradually increase the amount of clear fluids or rehydration fluids every two hours.
- Build up to a bland diet after 8 hours.
- If the symptoms get worse or other symptoms develop, **ring your GP.**

PART ⑥ Breathing problems

Asthma

For reasons we are not sure of, asthma is on the increase. Part of the problem may be pollution in our environment, particularly exhaust fumes. Thankfully deaths from asthma attacks are declining, but with around 2000 deaths each year, many in children, it should be taken very seriously. It can appear at any stage in life but is more common in children. Modern treatments will prevent or stop the vast majority of asthma attacks and it is rare in very young children. Most asthma sufferers simply have mild symptoms and may never suffer a serious attack.

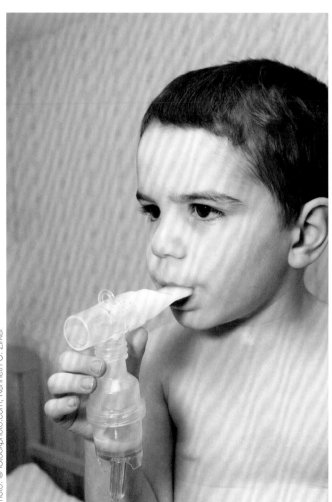

Photo: © iStockphoto.com, Kenneth C. Zirkel

Symptoms

The first sign of an attack can be as simple as a repeated cough, which can rapidly develop into a frightening breathlessness and tightness in the chest. This is usually painless, but after an attack there may be muscle strain which can ache. In the early stages a wheeze can be heard as the child breaths out. If they are suffering from a very serious attack there may be little or no wheeze or even the sound of breathing. They tend to sit up straight with their head slightly back with pursed lips. With severe attacks their lips may turn blue and they will be unable to speak. This is an emergency and you must dial 999/112.

Causes

Some forms of asthma are triggered (although not caused) by things like pollen, hay or house dust. Other forms seem to just happen with no apparent reason, although stress or a recent chest infection can act as triggers. Children who have hay fever or other allergies in the family are most likely to develop asthma.

Prevention

There is as yet no way of preventing the condition, but you can reduce the number and severity of attacks, particularly for a child with the allergic type of asthma. Keep a record of when and where they were with each attack. You may find it ties in with the presence of a particular pet, the pollen count on that day or even what they had to eat. Some of these things cannot be changed, but simple things like covering mattresses with a plastic cover to prevent dust mites, or keeping certain flowers out of the house, may make a difference. House dust mite faeces (droppings) are a powerful trigger for some asthma sufferers. Many vacuum cleaners can now be fitted with special filters which prevent these being blown into the air.

Complications

Badly-controlled asthma can be dangerous, especially if the early warning signs are ignored.

Treatment and self care

Nebulisers are sometimes supplied by the GP practice on a loan basis or from support groups. They can be useful for very young children who find hand-held inhalers difficult to use and can stop asthma attacks very rapidly. A device known as a spacer may also be used. In an emergency away from such machines, cut the large round end off a plastic lemonade bottle and fire the inhaler into the open end while the child breathes through the narrow screw-top hole.

Staying calm is vital when dealing with a child suffering an asthma attack. Remember the following points:
- Find their inhaler and help them use it.
- Dial 999/112 if it is a serious attack.
- Reassure them.
- Give them nothing to drink.
- Allow them to sit in any position they find most comfortable.
- Do not force them to lie down.
- If there is a nebuliser or spacer available, use it sooner rather than later.

Bronchiolitis

This condition of the lungs is very common and can lead to many hospital admissions. It is more common during the winter months and in boys. It mainly affects children up to two years old, with most cases happening at around six months old.

Cause

A virus called Respiratory Syncytial Virus (RSV) is often to blame (there is RSV positive and RSV negative bronchiolitis). It makes the small airways or bronchioles in the lungs narrow and fill with mucus, making breathing difficult. Although it usually lasts around seven days, it can also leave a lingering cough for weeks afterwards.

Signs and symptoms

An irritating cough is common but wheezing is usually the first sign. This obviously makes feeding more difficult for the baby. A fever is also often present. It is generally self-limiting and will clear up on its own, but you should ring your doctor if there is any sudden difficulty in breathing following a cough or cold, such as rapid breathing or wheezing, especially if there is also excessive drowsiness.

Treatment and self care

Admission to hospital is needed only in the most severe cases where the baby's breathing is badly affected and may require oxygen therapy and fluids.

Mild cases can be treated at home:

- Raise the head of the cot to make breathing easier at night.
- Hang damp towels on the radiator to raise the humidity in the nursery (but take care not to cause a fire hazard – check the radiator first. You may not be able to put anything on top of it). Alternatively, use a room humidifier, making sure it is out of the baby's reach.
- Make sure the baby is taking plenty of fluids.
- Nose drops can actually make things worse if you use them too often for too long. Take your doctor's advice on their use.

Choking

Choking happens surprisingly often. Immediate action is vital, so it is important to know the correct steps to follow:

- Check inside the mouth, and remove any obstruction.
- If you can't see or feel any obstruction, bend them over your hand or lap and give them 5 taps (not hard slaps) between their shoulder blades.
- If there is no response, turn them over and using two fingers only press firmly in their breast bone five times.
- If the blockage is not completely cleared, or the child continues to have trouble breathing, start again while someone seeks urgent medical attention.

Croup

Children between the ages of three months and six years are most likely to suffer from this condition which produces a seal-like barking cough which sounds terrible but is actually rarely serious. The symptoms usually lasts from three to seven days. As bad luck would have it, the cough is invariably worse during the night.

Causes
Thick mucus at the back of throat follows the initial viral infection.

Prevention
There is no known prevention for croup.

Self care
Croup can be treated by steam inhalation and does not need antibiotics. Stay calm. Getting upset will only make matters worse. If you have a bathroom, fill the bath with hot water so it steams. Alternatively run the shower on full heat with the shower door open. Otherwise choose a room which is safe to run a kettle to produce lots of steam. Simply sit with your child, allowing them to breath the warm steam in the room but not directly from the bath, shower or kettle.

Note
Inhaling a peanut or other small piece of food will produce the same kind of shortness of breath. If your child coughs and has a problem with their breathing while eating, take them to your hospital's Accident & Emergency department.

A serious but now very rare condition called epiglottitis (inflammation of the flap that closes the airway during swallowing) can be confused with croup. Fortunately the symptoms are not the same. Children with epiglottitis tend to drool while tilting their heads forward. They may have a fever and protrude their jaw as they try to breathe. Epiglottitis is caused by the same bacteria which causes one type of meningitis and has become less common since the introduction of the Hib vaccination, clearly showing the value of immunisations.

Croup can be treated by steam inhalation

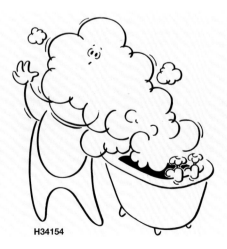

H34154

Breathing difficulties

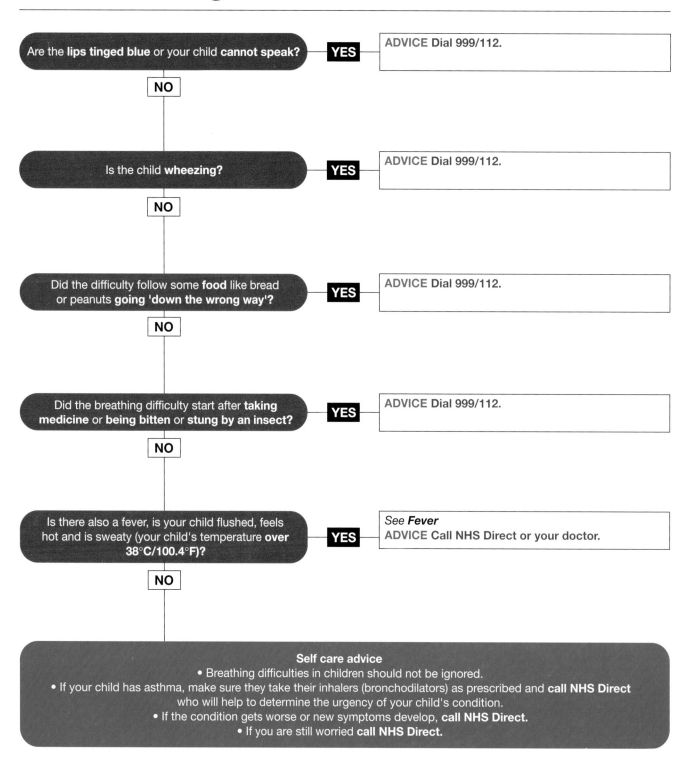

Are the **lips tinged blue** or your child **cannot speak?** — **YES** → ADVICE Dial 999/112.

NO

Is the child **wheezing?** — **YES** → ADVICE Dial 999/112.

NO

Did the difficulty follow some **food** like bread or peanuts **going 'down the wrong way'?** — **YES** → ADVICE Dial 999/112.

NO

Did the breathing difficulty start after **taking medicine** or **being bitten** or **stung by an insect?** — **YES** → ADVICE Dial 999/112.

NO

Is there also a fever, is your child flushed, feels hot and is sweaty (your child's temperature **over 38°C/100.4°F)?** — **YES** → *See **Fever*** ADVICE Call NHS Direct or your doctor.

NO

Self care advice
• Breathing difficulties in children should not be ignored.
• If your child has asthma, make sure they take their inhalers (bronchodilators) as prescribed and **call NHS Direct** who will help to determine the urgency of your child's condition.
• If the condition gets worse or new symptoms develop, **call NHS Direct.**
• If you are still worried **call NHS Direct.**

Coughing

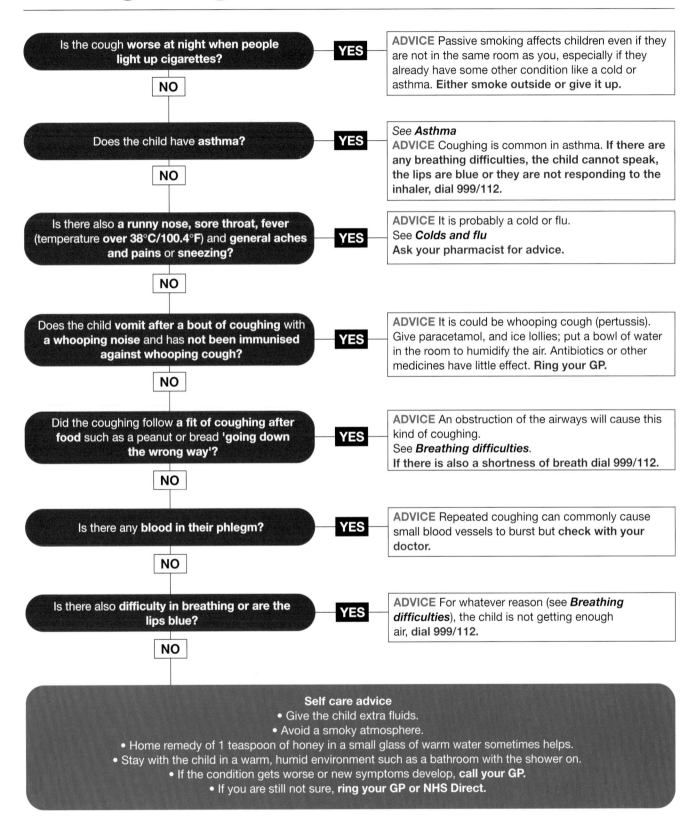

Is the cough **worse at night when people light up cigarettes?** — **YES**

ADVICE Passive smoking affects children even if they are not in the same room as you, especially if they already have some other condition like a cold or asthma. **Either smoke outside or give it up.**

NO

Does the child have **asthma?** — **YES**

See *Asthma*
ADVICE Coughing is common in asthma. **If there are any breathing difficulties, the child cannot speak, the lips are blue or they are not responding to the inhaler, dial 999/112.**

NO

Is there also **a runny nose, sore throat, fever** (temperature **over 38°C/100.4°F**) and **general aches and pains** or **sneezing?** — **YES**

ADVICE It is probably a cold or flu.
See *Colds and flu*
Ask your pharmacist for advice.

NO

Does the child **vomit after a bout of coughing** with **a whooping noise** and has **not been immunised against whooping cough?** — **YES**

ADVICE It is could be whooping cough (pertussis). Give paracetamol, and ice lollies; put a bowl of water in the room to humidify the air. Antibiotics or other medicines have little effect. **Ring your GP.**

NO

Did the coughing follow **a fit of coughing after food** such as a peanut or bread **'going down the wrong way'?** — **YES**

ADVICE An obstruction of the airways will cause this kind of coughing.
See *Breathing difficulties*.
If there is also a shortness of breath dial 999/112.

NO

Is there any **blood in their phlegm?** — **YES**

ADVICE Repeated coughing can commonly cause small blood vessels to burst but **check with your doctor.**

NO

Is there also **difficulty in breathing or are the lips blue?** — **YES**

ADVICE For whatever reason (see *Breathing difficulties*), the child is not getting enough air, **dial 999/112.**

NO

Self care advice
- Give the child extra fluids.
- Avoid a smoky atmosphere.
- Home remedy of 1 teaspoon of honey in a small glass of warm water sometimes helps.
- Stay with the child in a warm, humid environment such as a bathroom with the shower on.
- If the condition gets worse or new symptoms develop, **call your GP.**
- If you are still not sure, **ring your GP or NHS Direct.**

PART 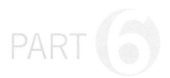 **6**

Skin problems

Bites and stings

Insects
Insect bites and stings can be painful but they are not usually serious, even in children. Most can be treated with simple, common-sense remedies without needing the attention of your doctor.

Causes
Midges, horse flies, bees, wasps, centipedes, ants, etc. The list is long, but thankfully there are no killers within the UK.

Symptoms
At first you may mistake the marks for something more serious. Looking very closely you may be able to see the small hole of the bite. The 'spot' is invariably itchy and may swell, particularly if it came from a horse fly (clegg).

Prevention
Insect repellents work. Use a mosquito net around the bed when in infested areas, particularly for children.

Treatment and self care
Although itchy and sometimes painful, insect bites and stings are rarely dangerous and need only some antihistamine or local anaesthetic cream from your pharmacist.

Initially, apply a cold compress to insect bites and stings. Remove bee stings with tweezers by gripping the base of the sting nearest to the skin to avoid squeezing the poison sac which may still contain some venom. Remove ticks by covering them with a smear of petroleum jelly, which blocks their breathing holes, and causes them to drop off. Simply pulling at the tick or trying to burn it off can leave the head in the skin, leading to infection.

Seek medical attention if:
- There is a known allergy to bites and stings.
- The sting or tick cannot be removed.
- There is infection around the site.
- There is a fever or shortness of breath.

Complications
Some children are strongly allergic to bites and stings and can be very ill. If there is any shortage of breath, dial 999/112. Bites can become infected by scratching.

Animals
Animal bites need urgent medical attention, as they may become infected if not treated. Small animal bites should be thoroughly cleaned with soap and water and covered with a sterile dressing. For serious bites, apply direct pressure with a clean cloth to control the bleeding and seek assistance.

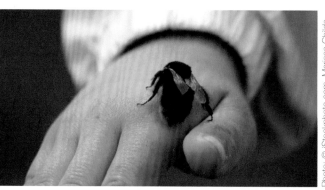

Photo: © iStockphoto.com, Marissa Childs

Eczema

This skin condition can vary from being merely a nuisance to posing serious risks to the baby or child. It is more common in children and is basically an inflammation of the skin producing dry flaky patches, usually on the inside of joints such as the elbow. It is normally a mild condition.

Symptoms

There are various types of eczema but in the baby the inherited form (atopic eczema) is the most common. Children with eczema tend also to suffer from allergies such as hay fever in later life. Seborrhoeic dermatitis is the name for eczema that affects the scalp, otherwise known as cradle cap, and this is not an indication of any future problems with allergies (see *Cradle cap* on page 164).

Causes

Unfortunately the cause is unknown, but it does tend to run in families.

Treatment

Keeping the skin moist with emollient ointments is important, and your doctor or pharmacist will advise you. Steroid creams can have a dramatic effect on the severe forms of eczema, not least in preventing scarring. Unfortunately they can make the skin more prone to infection and may cause thinning of the skin with constant use. Prolonged use with absorption of the steroid can also cause metabolic problems later in life. Only use them under your doctor's direction.

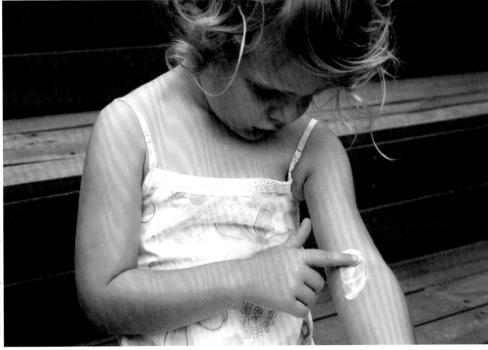

Photo: © iStockphoto.com, Steve Wilson

Lice

Wherever there is hair there can be lice and they have no respect for age when it comes to taking up squatters' rights. They are small, six-legged wingless insects, pin-head size when they hatch, less than match-head size when fully grown and grey/brown in colour. Nits are egg sacs, often empty, which hatch between 7 and 10 days after laying. Nits may still be found even after all the lice have been cleared. This doesn't necessarily mean there are live lice in the hair.

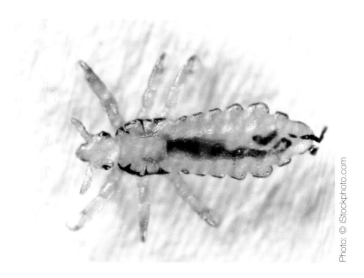

Symptoms

Lice are embarrassing but rarely if ever harmful. They do not suck blood, and the itchiness is often caused by small scratches on the scalp from over enthusiastic combing or finger nails.

Causes

Social status means nothing to lice, but they do seem to be more commonly found on children's scalps as they make intimate contact more often than adults. Although lice cannot fly, jump or swim, they are expert climbers and will cling on to any passing hair. They have a natural camouflage and can be difficult to detect, especially when there are only a few small lice present. It is almost impossible to prevent them amongst young children.

Treatment and self care

You can detect them by using a fine steel or plastic comb (from your pharmacist) on wet hair. This is helped by using a conditioner. Unless you actually detect living, moving lice you do not need to treat. There are several treatment options:

- Hair lotions using insecticides. You need to also check all close family/friends by the 'wet combing' method and treat anyone who is found to have lice at the same time, to prevent re-infection. Ensure you have enough lotion to treat all those affected and follow the instructions on the packet carefully.
- The 'Bug Busting' treatment method. This depends solely on physically removing any lice present. Success depends largely upon adopting a painstaking approach – as described in the Bug Busting kit available from some pharmacies, and by mail order from Community Hygiene Concern (see *Contacts* on page 193).
- The electric comb. Battery-powered, this is run through the child's hair and electrocutes any lice in its path, but not the child. As with bug busting, success depends on the thoroughness of the approach.

Insecticide lotion is probably more effective than bug busting, but there is increasing resistance to the insecticides, both by the lice who are becoming immune to their effects and by the parents who fear that repeated use may have a harmful effect on the child's nervous system.

Whatever method of control is adopted, it is easier to use on short hair.

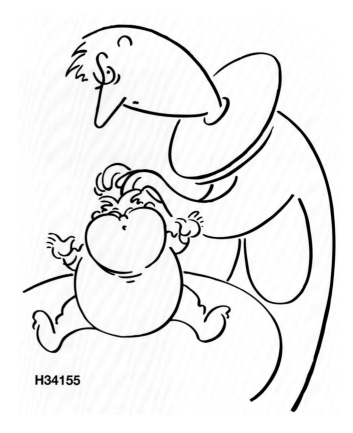

H34155

Sun burn

Although there is some controversy over the danger of exposure to too much sunlight, we do know that it can be harmful. Over the past few decades there has been a dramatic increase in the number of cases of malignant melanoma, a particularly nasty and potentially lethal skin cancer. Once considered rare, it is still increasing possibly due to the desire for sun drenched holidays. Australia has been in the forefront of educating people over the dangers of sunbathing.

Symptoms

Most people do not realise that they have badly burned themselves until later on in the day. The first sign of a burn is a reddening of the skin caused by blood vessels increasing in size to get rid of as much heat as possible. At this stage damage is already being done to the skin.

Causes

Ultra violet light (UV) can penetrate the outer layers of skin, especially in fair-skinned people. It heats and damages the lower layers causing skin loss. The body responds by increasing the amount of melanin, a black pigment, in the skin which prevents the sun from reaching the delicate lower skin layers.

Prevention

It's not too smart to be out in the sun wearing nothing but shorts, it's potentially deadly. Use a strong sun block (SPF 15 and over). Cover your child's body, especially the head, with appropriate clothing. Never leave a baby exposed to the sun, even if the weather is hazy.

Complications

If the exposure to the sun continues the skin will form blisters just as with a scald. These blisters burst very quickly and the covering skin is then lost exposing red skin beneath. If this is extensive, a large amount of body fluids can be lost; a particular danger to babies and small children who do not have a large body mass.

Like any burn, skin damaged by overexposure to UV can scar.

Long term exposure to the sun causes the collagen network within the skin to become less flexible. This makes the skin lose its elasticity so it droops, folds and wrinkles very easily.

Self care

A badly burnt baby or small child needs to go to hospital. Treat sun burn like any other burn. There are lotions you can apply which will ease the pain but they cannot prevent the damage which is already done. Give plenty of fluids and keep out of the sun for a few days. Use only tepid baths.

Note: There is no 'safe' exposure time. The rate at which you burn depends on the colour of your skin. Fair complexions are the easiest to damage with UV. Dark skin is the most resistant but will still be burned with prolonged exposure. Generally after 15 minutes on a first exposure white skin is already damaged.

Action

See your pharmacist.

Cuts and grazes

For a minor cut, press the wound with a clean fabric pad for a few minutes to help stop the bleeding. For a cut on an arm or leg, elevate the limb. Water may be used to wipe around the edge of the cut or graze. Once clean, apply a dressing such as a plaster.

Seek medical attention if:
● The cut is deep cut and the edges cannot be pulled together.
● Severe redness or swelling develops after a couple of days (this may be a sign of an infection).
● Severe bleeding from a wound needs immediate medical attention. While waiting for expert help, lie the child down and raise the injured part of the body above the level of the heart to help reduce blood loss. Place a clean cloth against the wound and press firmly. Secure this pad in place. Never use a tourniquet (something tied round the limb to stop the blood flow) - serious illness or even death can result from the blood clots which will form.

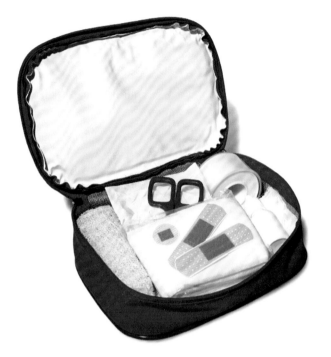

Photo: © iStockphoto.com, Luis C. Torres

Burns and scalds

Any burn or scald requires immediate action.

Remove tight clothing if possible. Cool the affected area with cold water for at least 10 minutes, then cover with a light, non-fluffy material. For a limb, kitchen film or a polythene bag may be used. Don't burst any blisters and don't apply any cream or ointments. (The exception is mild sunburn, which may be soothed with a lotion like calamine.)

Seek medical attention if:
● The burn is larger than the size of the child's hand.
● The burn is on the face.
● The skin is broken.

Severe burns need urgent medical attention. Cool the burn down, cover it with a sterile dressing, and get the child to your local accident and emergency department immediately or call for an ambulance. While waiting for the ambulance, make them lie down and raise their legs. This helps keep blood available for the vital organs. Don't remove clothes if they are sticking to the skin.

Cradle cap

A harmless scale which builds up on the scalp.

Symptoms
A thick white/yellow waxy scale builds up on the scalp. There is no bleeding or obvious irritation unless too vigorous attempts are made to remove it. There is no fever and the child is perfectly well.

Causes
Like many other forms of eczema (see page 161), the cause is unknown.

Prevention
Routine cleaning will prevent it in most cases.

Complications
There are no serious complications.

Self care
A form of eczema, it responds well to simply rubbing the affected parts of the scalp with olive oil. Leave it on overnight before washing it off with a mild shampoo in the morning.

Shampoos are available from your pharmacist, but you should try rubbing with olive oil first. Ask your pharmacist for advice.

Cold sores (herpes simplex)

Cold sores are common, tend to recur and can be very sore.

Symptoms

The corners of the mouth are the mainly affected areas with crusty, oozing blisters.

Causes

Herpes is a virus which lies dormant in nerve endings within the skin. The virus erupts during stress, use of steroids and for vague reasons such as sunlight exposure. There is a well-recognised pattern:

- A tingling, itchy feeling is usually felt just before the rash forms.
- Tiny blisters appear, usually where the lips join the skin.
- The blisters become sore and itchy.
- They then crust over and last about one week before disappearing.

Prevention and treatment

Herpes is highly infectious and can be passed on through kissing particularly while blisters are erupting. Babies tend to get kissed a great deal, so they are at risk of picking up a herpes simplex infection. People are at most risk of passing on an infection while the blisters are erupting so they should avoid kissing the baby during this time.

Paracetamol elixir helps with the pain, but for babies under 3 months use only under strict advice from your pharmacist or GP.

Lip salves can be applied before taking the baby into bright sunlight. The baby should also wear a hat.

There are topical medicines which limit the infection (ask your pharmacist).

Heat rash

All babies and children will have a rash at some time and these may sometimes be simply a 'heat rash'

Symptoms

It often looks like a fine pattern of tiny red spots which come and go but tend to disappear if their temperature is lowered.

The baby will be perfectly well with no other symptoms. A meningitis rash will not blanch when pressed with the side of a glass tumbler (see *Meningitis* on page 181).

Causes

A cold or other viral infection is the most common cause. Too many clothes or bedding will also cause it.

Prevention

If your baby gets too hot cool them down immediately by removing their clothes and keeping them in a cool room with tepid sponging. Keep an open mind, if things are getting worse call your doctor/999/112 (see *Rashes* on pages 168 to 170 and *Fever* on page 182).

Hives (urticaria)

Hives (urticaria or nettle rash) are small raised red spots, often itchy, which you can feel. They are rarely serious unless combined with any breathing problems. The rash will usually disappear in a few hours without any treatment.

Causes

It is most often caused by a viral infection but may be caused by certain foods and plants (eg, nettles).

Complications

Rarely the rash is severe and associated with breathing difficulties. This is an emergency so dial 999/112.

Treatment and care

Antihistamine creams and anti-histamine medicine may help. Ask your pharmacist.

If there is any shortness of breath dial 999/112.

Purpura

Serious problems are rare but these irregularly-shaped dark red spots could follow an allergic reaction to infection or some disorder of the blood.

Symptoms

The spots are not usually irritating, range from around pin-head size to a couple of centimetres (around one inch), tend to come and go and will not turn white (blanch) when pressed with a glass tumbler.

Causes

Children between 2 and 10 years are most likely to be affected. There are a number of causes, but anything that affects the ability of the blood to clot can cause this rash.

Treatment

Dial 999/112.

Nappy rash

Rashes in the nappy area are common but are not inevitable and can be reduced in severity or avoided completely.

Symptoms

The rash is usually red, not raised and confined to the nappy area.

Causes

Urine is highly irritant, especially in babies, as it contains ammonia. If it is cleaned away quickly enough, or the baby is allowed to have the nappy off for a while, the rash will not appear.

Prevention

As far as is possible, change each nappy immediately following soiling. Remember that urine can be every bit as irritating as faeces. Avoid disposable wipes containing alcohol (remember aftershaves after a bad shave? Same thing but on a far more sensitive surface than your chin) or moisturising chemicals. Instead use plenty of warm water. Leave the nappy off as much as is practical, particularly any plastic pants. Dry, cool skin rarely forms a nappy rash. Re-usable nappies should be washed as directed by the manufacturer. Avoid caustic household detergents which tend to leave residual traces no matter how well they are rinsed.

Complications

An angry red rash which does not respond or extends beyond the nappy area may be a fungal infection (candida). You need an anti-fungal cream and possibly an oral anti-fungal agent as it often starts in the mouth. Ask your pharmacist or doctor.

Self care

Promptly treat any rash appearing with ointment from your pharmacist.

Avoid talcum powder. It can cake badly and cause even more irritation.

Scabies

Although intensely itchy, scabies is rarely a serious condition.

Symptoms
Red lines which follow the burrows of the mite as it travels in the skin soon merge with the inevitable scratching. It is usually worse at night when the mite is most active.

Causes
Scabies is caused by a mite which burrows just under the skin, often between the fingers, on wrists, elbows and the genital areas causing a red rash. It can only come from contact with infected people.

Prevention
It is very difficult to prevent.

Complications
Bacterial infection from excessive scratching can make the situation worse.

Treatment and self care
Use lotions or creams which are available from your pharmacist over the counter or on prescription. All of the body will need to be covered with the ointment for 24 hours and all clothing and bedding should be washed thoroughly. All the family must also be treated. Use under strict advice from doctor or pharmacist.

'Slapped cheek' disease

Few conditions fit the name better. This is a mild illness characterised by a very vivid, red fiery rash on the cheeks, and a less intense rash on the arms and legs with occasional joint pains. It is also known as 'slapped cheek syndrome' and 'fifth disease'.

Cause
Despite the popular name (the formal name is erythema infectiosum), it is not caused by abuse but by infection with a virus called Human Parvovirus B19.

Treatment and self care
Generally it is self-limiting and will disappear on its own but you can make life more pleasant for the baby with some simple treatments:
- Sponge the baby with tepid water, all over. By allowing body heat to dry the skin rather than towelling it dry the baby will cool down quickly and feel much better.
- Sugar-free paracetamol syrup helps to help reduce fever and eases aches and pains. Take careful note of the dose on the bottle.
- Don't put too many clothes on them. No clothes at all in a warm room is best.
- Keep the fluids up, they will lose water through a fever.

Infant rashes

Is the rash a crusty white scale on the scalp? — **YES**

See *Cradle cap*
ADVICE Cradle cap is a form of eczema, it responds well to simply rubbing the affected parts of the scalp with olive oil. Leave it on over night before washing it off with a mild shampoo in the morning. **See your pharmacist.**

NO

Is there a fever (the temperature is over 38°C/100.4°F)? — **YES**

See *Rashes with fever*

NO

Is the rash mainly in the nappy area? — **YES**

See *Nappy rash*
ADVICE Rashes in the nappy area are common but can be reduced in severity or avoided completely.
• As far as possible, change each nappy following soiling.
• As much as possible, leave the nappy off, particularly any plastic pants. Dry cool skin rarely forms a nappy rash.
• An angry red rash which won't respond or extends beyond the nappy area may be a fungal infection (Candida). **Ask your pharmacist or doctor.**

NO

Is the rash red, itchy, flaky and in more than one place? — **YES**

See *Eczema*
ADVICE Eczema covers a range of skin problems. There is a wide range of products which will help stop the itchiness and keep the skin moist. Follow your doctor's advice on the use of topical steroid creams. Call NHS Direct, **but call your doctor if:**
• The eczema is spreading very quickly.
• The skin is becoming infected.
• There is severe pain.

NO

Is the rash blotchy red and difficult to feel? — **YES**

See *Heat rash*
ADVICE All babies and children will have a heat rash at some time. No treatment is required other than lowering their temperature by moving them from the heat, removing their clothes and keeping them in a cool room.

NO

Is the rash dark red, mainly on the elbows, legs, buttocks and does it change its appearance and place on the skin? — **YES**

See *Purpura*
ADVICE Serious problems are rare but these irregularly shaped dark red spots could follow an allergic reaction to infection or some disorder of the blood. **Stop answering the questions and call NHS Direct.**

NO

Self care advice
• A rash alone is unlikely to be serious.
• Encourage the child to rest and observe closely for signs of illness.
• Ensure the child is drinking plenty of fluids.
• Paracetamol may be helpful if the child is restless.
• Antihistamine cream may provide some relief - a pharmacist will be able to advise you further.
• Calamine lotion will give relief for a short time.
• 2 tablespoons of sodium bicarbonate added to bath water may relieve any itching.
• If the condition gets worse or if any other symptoms develop **call NHS Direct.**

Itchy rashes

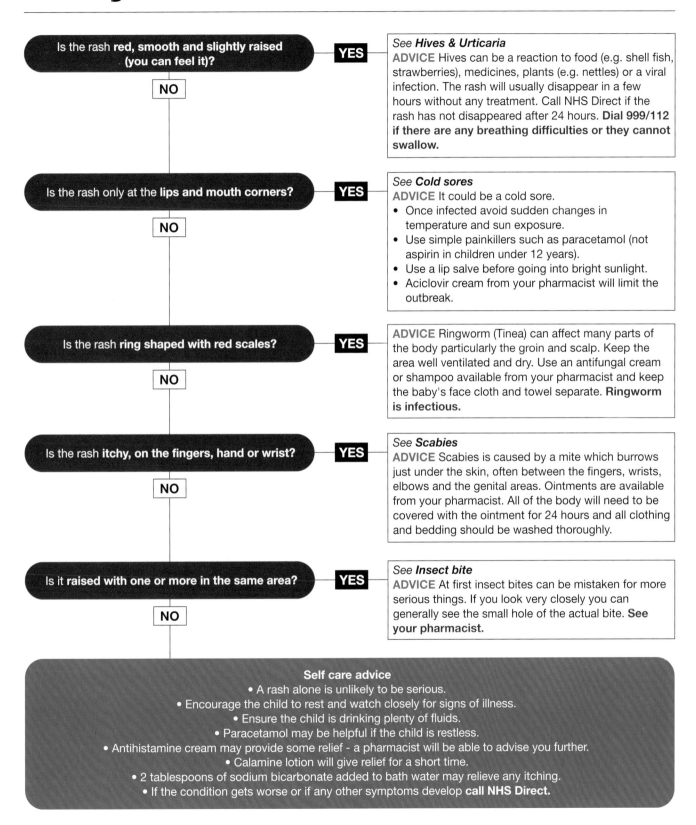

Is the rash red, smooth and slightly raised (you can feel it)? — **YES**

See ***Hives & Urticaria***
ADVICE Hives can be a reaction to food (e.g. shell fish, strawberries), medicines, plants (e.g. nettles) or a viral infection. The rash will usually disappear in a few hours without any treatment. Call NHS Direct if the rash has not disappeared after 24 hours. **Dial 999/112 if there are any breathing difficulties or they cannot swallow.**

NO

Is the rash only at the lips and mouth corners? — **YES**

See ***Cold sores***
ADVICE It could be a cold sore.
- Once infected avoid sudden changes in temperature and sun exposure.
- Use simple painkillers such as paracetamol (not aspirin in children under 12 years).
- Use a lip salve before going into bright sunlight.
- Aciclovir cream from your pharmacist will limit the outbreak.

NO

Is the rash ring shaped with red scales? — **YES**

ADVICE Ringworm (Tinea) can affect many parts of the body particularly the groin and scalp. Keep the area well ventilated and dry. Use an antifungal cream or shampoo available from your pharmacist and keep the baby's face cloth and towel separate. **Ringworm is infectious.**

NO

Is the rash itchy, on the fingers, hand or wrist? — **YES**

See ***Scabies***
ADVICE Scabies is caused by a mite which burrows just under the skin, often between the fingers, wrists, elbows and the genital areas. Ointments are available from your pharmacist. All of the body will need to be covered with the ointment for 24 hours and all clothing and bedding should be washed thoroughly.

NO

Is it raised with one or more in the same area? — **YES**

See ***Insect bite***
ADVICE At first insect bites can be mistaken for more serious things. If you look very closely you can generally see the small hole of the actual bite. **See your pharmacist.**

NO

Self care advice
- A rash alone is unlikely to be serious.
- Encourage the child to rest and watch closely for signs of illness.
- Ensure the child is drinking plenty of fluids.
- Paracetamol may be helpful if the child is restless.
- Antihistamine cream may provide some relief - a pharmacist will be able to advise you further.
- Calamine lotion will give relief for a short time.
- 2 tablespoons of sodium bicarbonate added to bath water may relieve any itching.
- If the condition gets worse or if any other symptoms develop **call NHS Direct.**

Rashes with fever

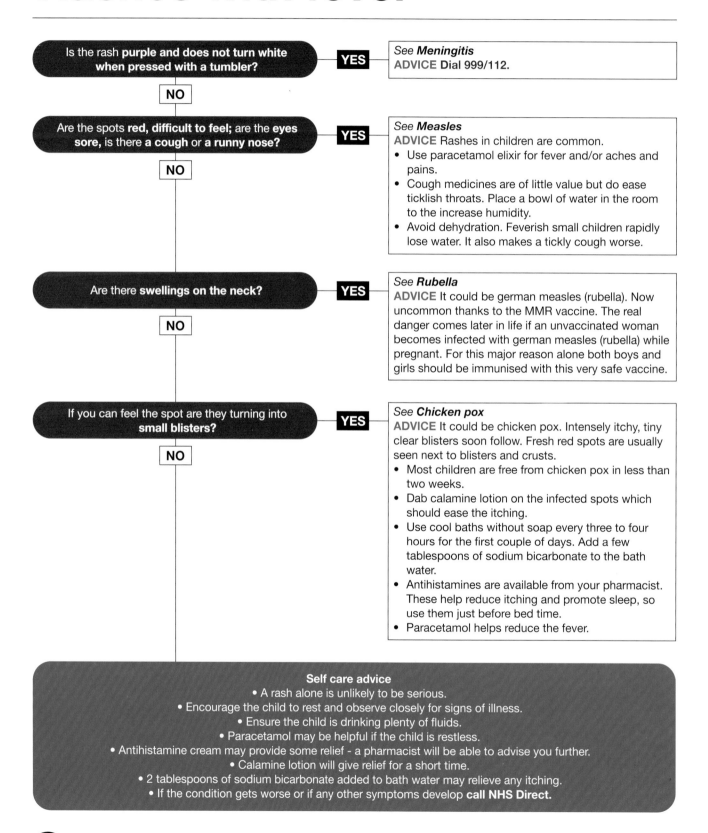

Is the rash **purple and does not turn white when pressed with a tumbler?**

YES → See *Meningitis*
ADVICE Dial 999/112.

NO

Are the spots **red, difficult to feel; are the eyes sore,** is there **a cough** or **a runny nose?**

YES → See *Measles*
ADVICE Rashes in children are common.
- Use paracetamol elixir for fever and/or aches and pains.
- Cough medicines are of little value but do ease ticklish throats. Place a bowl of water in the room to the increase humidity.
- Avoid dehydration. Feverish small children rapidly lose water. It also makes a tickly cough worse.

NO

Are there **swellings on the neck?**

YES → See *Rubella*
ADVICE It could be german measles (rubella). Now uncommon thanks to the MMR vaccine. The real danger comes later in life if an unvaccinated woman becomes infected with german measles (rubella) while pregnant. For this major reason alone both boys and girls should be immunised with this very safe vaccine.

NO

If you can feel the spot are they turning into **small blisters?**

YES → See *Chicken pox*
ADVICE It could be chicken pox. Intensely itchy, tiny clear blisters soon follow. Fresh red spots are usually seen next to blisters and crusts.
- Most children are free from chicken pox in less than two weeks.
- Dab calamine lotion on the infected spots which should ease the itching.
- Use cool baths without soap every three to four hours for the first couple of days. Add a few tablespoons of sodium bicarbonate to the bath water.
- Antihistamines are available from your pharmacist. These help reduce itching and promote sleep, so use them just before bed time.
- Paracetamol helps reduce the fever.

NO

Self care advice
- A rash alone is unlikely to be serious.
- Encourage the child to rest and observe closely for signs of illness.
- Ensure the child is drinking plenty of fluids.
- Paracetamol may be helpful if the child is restless.
- Antihistamine cream may provide some relief - a pharmacist will be able to advise you further.
- Calamine lotion will give relief for a short time.
- 2 tablespoons of sodium bicarbonate added to bath water may relieve any itching.
- If the condition gets worse or if any other symptoms develop **call NHS Direct.**

PART 6 **Bones and joints**

Broken bones and dislocations

Broken bones and dislocations always need immediate medical attention. They can be very painful, and you can help by reassuring the child and keeping them still.

Broken limbs

Steady and support the limb with your hands. If a leg is broken, place padding around it to prevent movement. A broken arm or collar bone should be supported on the affected side to the body.

Injured neck or spine

Keep the injured child as still as possible without heavily restraining them. It is essential not to move someone with a neck or spine injury unless they are in imminent danger of further injury. If the casualty becomes unconscious, carefully place them in recovery position while keeping the spine in line at all times.

Dislocated joints

Never try to force a joint back into place. Simply support the limb and seek emergency help.

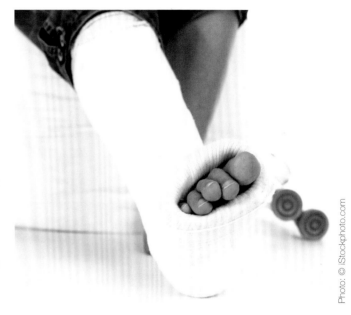

Photo: © iStockphoto.com

Sprains, strains and bruising

Remember 'RICE' (Rest, Ice, Compress, Elevation).
- Rest the injured part as much as possible.
- Immediately after the injury, pack the area with ice wrapped in a cloth – a bag of frozen peas works well – to reduce swelling. Keep the ice in place for about 10 minutes.
- Gently compress the injury and bind the area with an elastic bandage so it is well supported, but make sure you doesn't restrict blood flow.
- To minimise swelling, keep the injured part elevated as much of the time as possible.
  Seek medical attention if:
- You think there may be a broken bone – immobilise the area with padding and seek aid immediately.
- Symptoms don't improve.
- Bruising remains after several days.

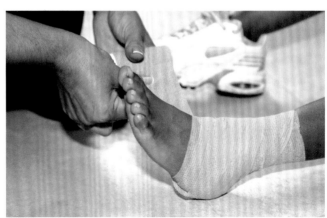

Don't bind the injury too tight

Photo: © iStockphoto.com

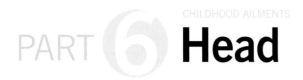

Head

Nose bleeds

Nose bleeds are common and most are easily dealt with. Sit the child down, leaning slightly forward, and tell them to breathe through the mouth. Then pinch the nose firmly for about 10 minutes. Seek medical help if the bleeding continues for more than 30 minutes or if you suspect the nose is broken.

Oral thrush

Contrary to common thought, thrush is not caused by bacteria or viruses. It is candida albicans, a yeast fungus, which causes the problem. For some reason it is most common young children and babies, even though there is often no apparent reason for it to grow. It can also be encouraged by repeated courses of antibiotics or steroids.

Symptoms

Sore, creamy yellow patches on the inner cheeks and throat. These turn into a nasty raw looking area when rubbed. Babies can have difficulty feeding and may cry, particularly if drinking fruit juice.

Causes

Oral thrush is very common in babies and there is often no obvious cause, other than (if applicable) repeated antibiotic or steroid treatments.

Prevention

Although bottle feeding is not a direct cause provided the equipment is properly sterilised, breastfeeding may give a degree of protection from infections generally.

Treatment

A course of antifungal drops will generally clear the infection quickly, but it can recur. If it does, you should seek medical advice.

Sticky eye

Soon after birth, babies can develop a discharge from one or both eyes which causes the eye lids to stick together. It can be caused by an infection picked up during birth. Gentle bathing with cotton wool soaked in tepid water will generally clear the problem. Blocked tear ducts can cause a similar appearance, although then there tends also to be tears running down their cheeks (see *Blocked tear ducts* on page 174).

A sticky eye which is also red in older babies and children is more likely to be conjunctivitis caused by a bacterial or viral infection that affects the lining of the outer membrane of the eye and the lids. It commonly affects both eyes at the same time.

Treatment and self care
- Gently bathe the affected eye with clean cotton wool soaked in cooled, tepid, boiled water.
- Throw away the cotton wool after each wipe.
- Wipe from the inner eyelid outwards.
- Do not share towels or flannels with other members of the family as conjunctivitis can be very infectious.
- Make an appointment to see your doctor if both eyes are infected or they don't clear up in a few days.

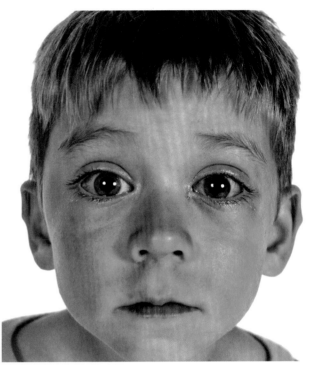

Photo: © iStockphoto.com, Jason Lugo

Blood in the white of the eye (subconjunctival haemorrhage)

A thin transparent layer covers the white of the eye called the conjunctiva. Bright red blood over the conjunctiva can be quite alarming yet it is generally completely harmless and very common, and parents worry unnecessarily that the child may have been hit or dropped. Tiny blood vessels beneath the protective layer (conjunctiva) burst and a small amount of blood is trapped under the conjunctiva.

Symptoms
The blood appears very quickly. Generally the blood will be over one part of the white of the eye but sometimes may cover most or all of it. The conjunctiva is tethered down in a ring around the transparent very front of the eye, the cornea. Blood can travel freely under the conjunctiva but not over the cornea itself.

Causes
It is common in babies and children when they cry for long periods.

Complications
Within a week or so it should disappear altogether.

Action
Unless there was trauma involved there is no need for a medical examination as the blood will gradually disperse on its own.

Blocked tear ducts

It's not a well-known fact, but newborn babies don't usually shed tears when they cry, this tends to happen a bit later in life. Even without crying there is always tear fluid running on to the surface of the eye to provide oxygen and nutrients, as the very front of the eye (the cornea) has no blood vessels. Watery eyes can therefore be caused by this tear fluid failing to drain away through the tear ducts at the nose side of each eye (this is why your nose 'runs' when you cry hard). Blocked tear ducts which have yet to open properly are a common cause, but a bacterial or viral infection (see *Sticky eye* on page 173) can also be a cause and is usually accompanied by a sticky discharge and redness around the eyes.

Treatment
If it is not settling, or there is also a 'sticky eye' or red eye, ask your doctor's advice.

Your health visitor can show you how to massage the area gently to help clear any blockage.

Always bathe the eye from the nose side outwards, using a fresh clean piece of cotton wool soaked in cooled boiled water each time. Do not use the same bit twice. Wash your hands before and afterwards and use a separate towel or flannel if there is any sign of infection, as it is highly contagious.

Cleft lip and palate

Times change. Cleft lip and palate were once the subject of myth, fear and abuse. Not only are abnormalities infinitely more acceptable in modern society, we now have the ability to treat them often very successfully. Just as well, as about one child in 1000 will be affected, not common but then not very rare either. The upper lip may have a defect which may be no more than a small notch, or which may extend right up to join one nostril. A gap in the roof of the mouth, cleft palate, may partially or completely divide it. Sometimes there are two gaps in the upper lip, extending up to both nostrils, and these may be associated with partial or complete cleft palate. Alternatively there may be only a cleft palate on its own, without any lip defect.

Symptoms

Unlike some congenital abnormalities, such as those affecting the heart, a cleft lip is often obvious. This is actually an advantage as it can then be recognised and steps taken early to rectify the situation. Feeding problems can often arise but in most cases these can be overcome with either bottle feeding or breastfeeding with a nipple shield which seals the area around the nipple, allowing the baby to suckle.

Causes

Facial development in the womb is incredibly complex with various parts needing to fuse along the mid-line. Any failure to join properly can cause a cleft lip or palate. Myths surround the whole area of cleft lip, most designed to make the parent feel as guilty and dreadful as possible. In truth we don't know the underlying cause although it may be possible to reduce the risk.

Diagnosis

Generally it is the parent, often the mother, who realises there is a problem. Sometimes a cleft palate will go unnoticed for longer until feeding becomes a problem. Referral to a surgeon specialising in this area will establish the extent of the problem and all children will benefit from modern surgery.

Prevention

There is no definitive way of prevention but it makes sense to follow guidelines on vitamin supplements, avoiding drugs, tobacco and alcohol during pregnancy.

Complications

Feeding is not a serious problem in almost all cases, but speech development can be affected unless early intervention takes place. This has major implications for the child's education. It's worth saying it again that modern surgery really can and does make a major change in the situation so there is no need for despondency.

Treatment

The surgical management of these conditions has improved greatly in recent decades and it is now rare to see the obvious deformity, called 'hare lip', resulting from treatment of a cleft lip. Good surgical repair is possible, usually between three months and one year of age.

   Treatment of cleft palate begins immediately after birth. A small device called a palatal obturator is used to cover the opening to help the baby to feed. There is often a team involved which includes surgeons, speech therapists, physiotherapists and dentists.

Earache

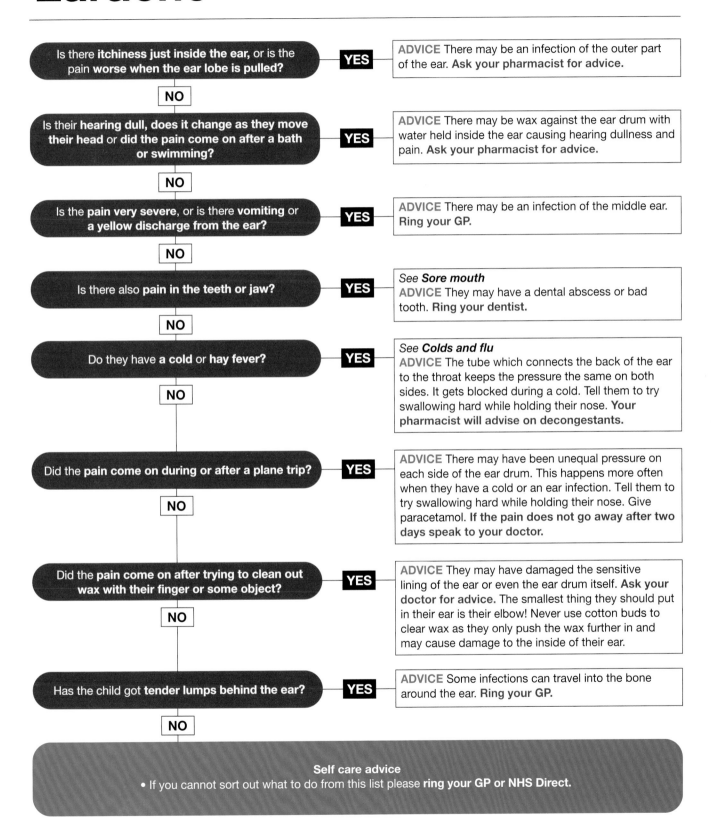

Is there **itchiness just inside the ear,** or is the pain **worse when the ear lobe is pulled?**

YES — ADVICE There may be an infection of the outer part of the ear. **Ask your pharmacist for advice.**

NO

Is their **hearing dull, does it change as they move their head** or did the pain come on after a bath or swimming?

YES — ADVICE There may be wax against the ear drum with water held inside the ear causing hearing dullness and pain. **Ask your pharmacist for advice.**

NO

Is the **pain very severe,** or is there **vomiting** or a yellow discharge from the ear?

YES — ADVICE There may be an infection of the middle ear. **Ring your GP.**

NO

Is there also **pain in the teeth or jaw?**

YES — See **Sore mouth**
ADVICE They may have a dental abscess or bad tooth. **Ring your dentist.**

NO

Do they have **a cold** or **hay fever?**

YES — See **Colds and flu**
ADVICE The tube which connects the back of the ear to the throat keeps the pressure the same on both sides. It gets blocked during a cold. Tell them to try swallowing hard while holding their nose. **Your pharmacist will advise on decongestants.**

NO

Did the **pain come on during or after a plane trip?**

YES — ADVICE There may have been unequal pressure on each side of the ear drum. This happens more often when they have a cold or an ear infection. Tell them to try swallowing hard while holding their nose. Give paracetamol. **If the pain does not go away after two days speak to your doctor.**

NO

Did the **pain come on after trying to clean out wax with their finger or some object?**

YES — ADVICE They may have damaged the sensitive lining of the ear or even the ear drum itself. **Ask your doctor for advice.** The smallest thing they should put in their ear is their elbow! Never use cotton buds to clear wax as they only push the wax further in and may cause damage to the inside of their ear.

NO

Has the child got **tender lumps behind the ear?**

YES — ADVICE Some infections can travel into the bone around the ear. **Ring your GP.**

NO

Self care advice
• If you cannot sort out what to do from this list please **ring your GP or NHS Direct.**

175

Head injury

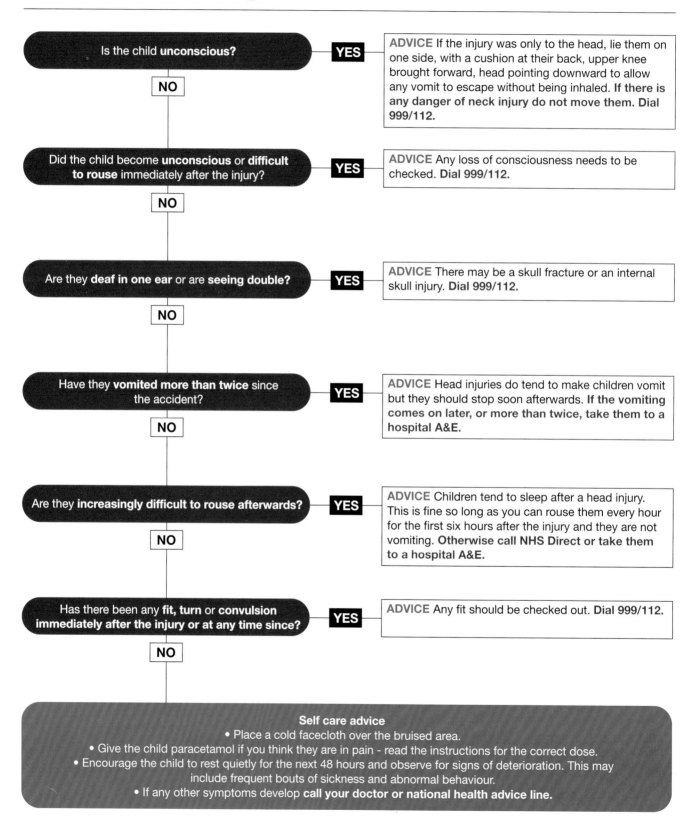

Is the child **unconscious?**

NO

YES — **ADVICE** If the injury was only to the head, lie them on one side, with a cushion at their back, upper knee brought forward, head pointing downward to allow any vomit to escape without being inhaled. **If there is any danger of neck injury do not move them. Dial 999/112.**

Did the child become **unconscious** or **difficult to rouse** immediately after the injury?

NO

YES — **ADVICE** Any loss of consciousness needs to be checked. **Dial 999/112.**

Are they **deaf in one ear** or are **seeing double?**

NO

YES — **ADVICE** There may be a skull fracture or an internal skull injury. **Dial 999/112.**

Have they **vomited more than twice** since the accident?

NO

YES — **ADVICE** Head injuries do tend to make children vomit but they should stop soon afterwards. **If the vomiting comes on later, or more than twice, take them to a hospital A&E.**

Are they **increasingly difficult to rouse afterwards?**

NO

YES — **ADVICE** Children tend to sleep after a head injury. This is fine so long as you can rouse them every hour for the first six hours after the injury and they are not vomiting. **Otherwise call NHS Direct or take them to a hospital A&E.**

Has there been any **fit, turn** or **convulsion** immediately after the injury or at any time since?

NO

YES — **ADVICE** Any fit should be checked out. **Dial 999/112.**

Self care advice
- Place a cold facecloth over the bruised area.
- Give the child paracetamol if you think they are in pain - read the instructions for the correct dose.
- Encourage the child to rest quietly for the next 48 hours and observe for signs of deterioration. This may include frequent bouts of sickness and abnormal behaviour.
- If any other symptoms develop **call your doctor or national health advice line.**

Sore mouth

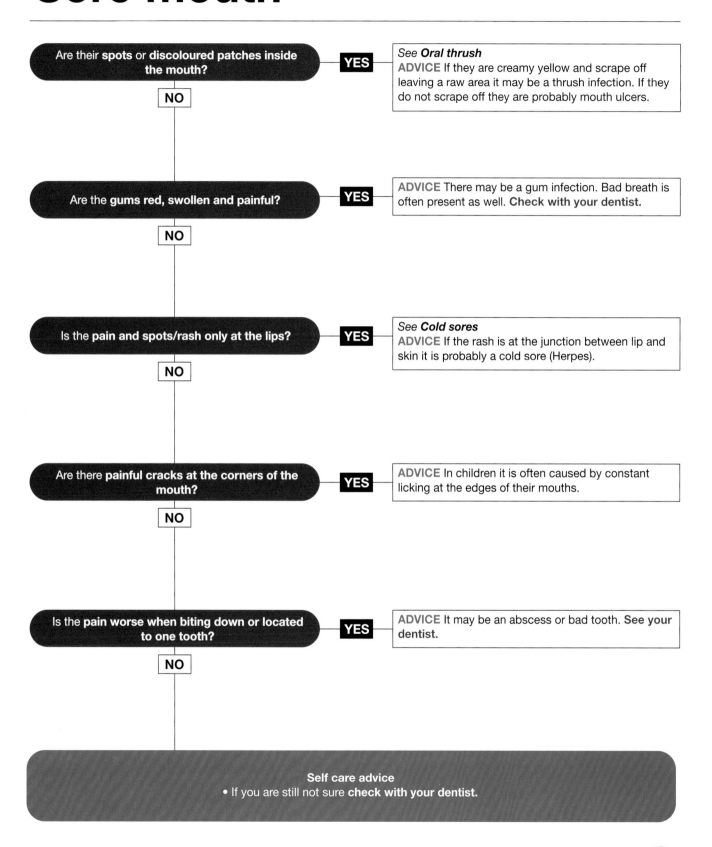

Are their spots or discoloured patches inside the mouth?

YES → See **Oral thrush**
ADVICE If they are creamy yellow and scrape off leaving a raw area it may be a thrush infection. If they do not scrape off they are probably mouth ulcers.

NO

Are the gums red, swollen and painful?

YES → ADVICE There may be a gum infection. Bad breath is often present as well. **Check with your dentist.**

NO

Is the pain and spots/rash only at the lips?

YES → See **Cold sores**
ADVICE If the rash is at the junction between lip and skin it is probably a cold sore (Herpes).

NO

Are there painful cracks at the corners of the mouth?

YES → ADVICE In children it is often caused by constant licking at the edges of their mouths.

NO

Is the pain worse when biting down or located to one tooth?

YES → ADVICE It may be an abscess or bad tooth. **See your dentist.**

NO

Self care advice
• If you are still not sure **check with your dentist.**

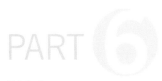

Infectious diseases

Chicken pox

The incubation period (the time from contact with the virus and onset of symptoms) is between 7 to 21 days. In most cases there are no symptoms before the rash appears. It is one of the more harmless infections.

Symptoms

A mild fever, stomach ache and a general feeling of being unwell can occur a day or two before the flat, red rash appears. This generally begins on the scalp, face and back, but can spread to any body surface although it is rarely seen on the palms of the hands or soles of the feet.

- Intensely itchy, tiny clear blisters full of virus particles then appear.
- New blisters appear as fresh red spots, usually seen next to old blisters and crusts.
- It generally takes less than two weeks to clear.

Causes

Chicken pox is a highly infectious virus and spreads quickly, especially between children. Close contact is all that is required to pass on the infection.

Prevention

There is no vaccine licensed in this country at present. Some parents advocate 'pox parties' to get the child infected at an early age. This is probably not wise, as there is no guarantee of infection in later life.

Complications

Thankfully, complications are very rare in children. There are reported cases of encephalitis (inflammation of the brain), meningitis or pneumonia but they are extremely rare.

More serious complications are seen in children who are taking medicines such as steroids as they can lower the body's immune defence system, or who have a medical condition which lowers their natural resistance.

Self care

- A few teaspoons of sodium bicarbonate in a cool bath can help relieve the itch.
- There are products available from your pharmacist to provide temporary relief.
- Calamine lotion is a traditional treatment to stop the itching. Put some in a spray bottle (as used on plants) and spray the child whilst stood in the bath or shower. The droplets so created cool the blisters and soothe quickly.
- Cotton socks on inquisitive hands will prevent too much scratching which can lead to infection.
- Paracetamol elixir helps reduce the fever. Do not give aspirin to children under 16 years of age.
- Ice lollies help lower temperature, provide sugar and water and at the same time reduce the irritation of mouth infection. They may be used in children over 4 years old.

More information

Chicken pox is no longer infectious 5 days after the blisters first appear or when all the blisters have scabbed over, whichever comes first.

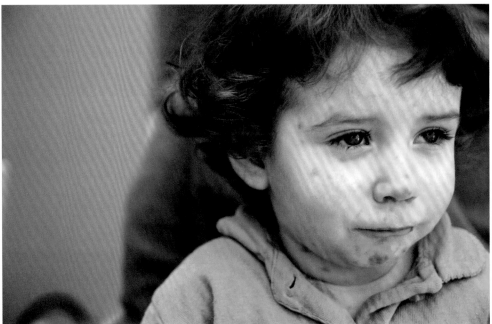

Measles

Young children are most vulnerable to this highly contagious viral infection. The 'triple vaccine' MMR (mumps, measles, rubella) vaccination programme made measles very rare in the UK, but it has now made an unwelcome return as vaccination rates have fallen in response to fears amongst parents over highly-publicised but un-substantiated links with autism and Crohn's disease.

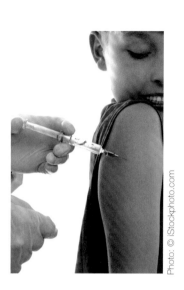

Symptoms
There is generally a pattern which is easy to recognise:
- Red eyes and sensitivity to light.
- Tiredness and general fatigue.
- Loss of appetite.
- Running nose and sneezing.
- A temperature of around 39°C (102.2°F).
- Irritable dry cough.
- Tiny white spots in the mouth and throat.
- A blotchy red rash that starts behind the ears, spreads to the face and then to the rest of the body and lasts for up to seven days.

Transmission
There is an incubation period (the time the disease takes to show after initial infection) of around 10 to 12 days. Physical contact, sneezing and clothing contaminated with nasal secretions all help to spread the infection.

Prevention
Vaccination is the best way but once a child has had measles they are also immune.

Complications
There are rare but serious complications from measles such as meningitis and pneumonia. More commonly, eyes and ears develop secondary infection which may need antibiotic treatment.

Treatment and self care
There is no cure for measles so once the rash starts it is a matter of treating the symptoms.
- Use a ball of damp cotton wool to clean away any crustiness around the eyes.
- Draw the curtains or blinds to ease their eyes from bright sunlight.
- Although cough medicines are of little proven value they may ease ticklish throats, but also try placing a bowl of water in the room.
- High temperature, aches and pains can be treated with paracetamol elixir.
- Feverish small children dehydrate very quickly which can make their cough worse. Keep up their fluids.
  Ideally, you should keep your child away from others for at least 7 days after the start of the rash, easier said than done.
  After four days the child usually feels better.

Colds and flu

Most of us can't tell the difference between a bad cold and flu, so you will be delighted to hear that most doctors can't either. The problem with children is they look so awful when it is just a bad cold. Even so, there are easy and effective ways to treat your child's colds and flu symptoms at home and with medicines from your pharmacy.

How to treat cold and flu symptoms:

● Get them to drink plenty of fluids.
● Use paracetamol (Calpol) according to the instructions (don't give aspirin to a child under 16 years because of the danger of its link with Reye's Syndrome). This will ease their sore throat and muscle aches while bringing their temperature down. Always take the suggested dosage for all medications.
● Don't encourage strenuous exercise, but at the same time it is often better if they sit up and watch TV rather than overheating in a bed. You can also keep a better eye on them.
● Encourage them to cover their mouth when they cough and sneeze.
● Wash your hands regularly as the virus is passed through skin contact.
● Keep the bedroom well-ventilated.
● If they do have flu let them take it easy.

You should contact your GP or ring NHS Direct (0845 464 7) if they are experiencing severe or prolonged symptoms, shortness of breath or are coughing up blood or phlegm (see *Fever* on page 182).

Antibiotics

Some people expect their GP to always give antibiotics to treat children's colds and flu symptoms. Colds and flu are viral illnesses. Antibiotics do not work on viral illness and in fact they can do more harm than good.

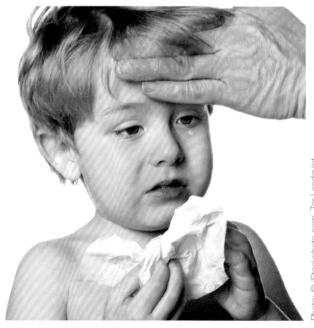

Photo: © iStockphoto.com, Tor Londqvist

Meningitis/septicaemia

Although a rare illness, this causes an inflammation of the brain lining which can be fatal, so it is rightly seen as a real threat by parents. Unfortunately the symptoms can be easily be mistaken for flu or a bad cold. Worse still, it is more difficult to be certain with babies and young children. If you are not sure, you must call your doctor/999/112.

Hib immunisation has reduced the number of people suffering from some types of meningitis/septicaemia. Unfortunately, we do not have vaccines for every type of meningitis/septicaemia, so we all still need to watch out for the symptoms.

Symptoms
Babies under 2 years may show:
● A difficulty to wake.
● A cry which may be high-pitched and different from normal.
● Vomiting repeatedly, not just after feeds.
● Refusing feeds, either from the bottle, breast or by spoon.
● Skin which may appear pale or blotchy, possibly with a red/purple rash which does not fade when you press a tumbler glass or a finger against the rash.
● The soft spot on top of your baby's head (the fontanelle) may be tight or bulging.
● The baby may seem irritable and dislike being handled.
● The body may be floppy or else stiff with jerky movements.
Remember, a fever may not be present in the early stages, and the symptoms can appear in any order. Not all babies show all of these signs.

Causes
Meningitis can be caused by either bacteria or viruses; in most cases bacterial causes are more serious.

Prevention
Vaccination for meningitis C for children and young people up to 17 years of age is safe and extremely effective. Some forms of meningitis do not, as yet, have a vaccination so the disease can still occur. It pays to keep an open mind when faced with puzzling signs of infection. Always call your GP/999/112 if you are concerned that things are not getting better.

People who have been in contact with someone who has had meningitis should contact a close relative of the patient to find out any instructions that they may have been given. Otherwise your doctor will be able to give you appropriate advice. Only those who have been in very close contact with the infected person (referred to as 'kissing contacts') are given antibiotics and vaccination.

German measles (rubella)

This once common and highly infections condition is now uncommon thanks to the MMR vaccine. Even so, with the confusion over the triple vaccine (MMR) the number of childhood cases is steadily rising.

Symptoms
The child is rarely ill but will have a mildly raised temperature and swollen glands on the neck and base of the skull.

The pin-head sized flat, red spots last around two days and need no treatment other than possibly some paracetamol for the slight fever.

Causes
The virus is very contagious and will spread quickly in a population which is not immune.

Prevention
Vaccination for girls and boys is both safe and effective.

Complications
Very rarely the virus that causes German measles (rubella) will cause an inflammation of the brain (encephalitis).

The real danger comes in later life if an unvaccinated woman becomes infected with German measles (rubella) while pregnant. For this major reason alone both boys and girls should be immunised.

Treatment and self care
Paracetamol will reduce the mild fever.

Roseola

This common condition is also known as 'fourth disease' and 'three-day fever'. It is more common in babies under one year old. Generally it shows itself with a high fever which lasts for around three or four days. As the fever drops, a rose-coloured, fine, flat, red spotty rash appears on the trunk. This spreads and then fades within 24 hours. Measles may first come to mind, but unlike measles the rash appears on the trunk first.

Treatment and self care
There is no 'cure', but it is almost always a mild condition which needs only simple care as for any fever:
● Sponge the baby with tepid water, all over. Allow the body heat to dry the skin rather than towelling it dry as it takes off the body heat as the water evaporates. This can be repeated as often as necessary.
● Regular doses of sugar-free paracetamol syrup help reduce fever and combat aches and pains, but take great care to use according to the manufacturer's instructions. If you are not sure, ask your pharmacist.
● Take their clothes off. In a warm room the baby needs only a tee shirt.
● Keep up with the fluids.

Fever

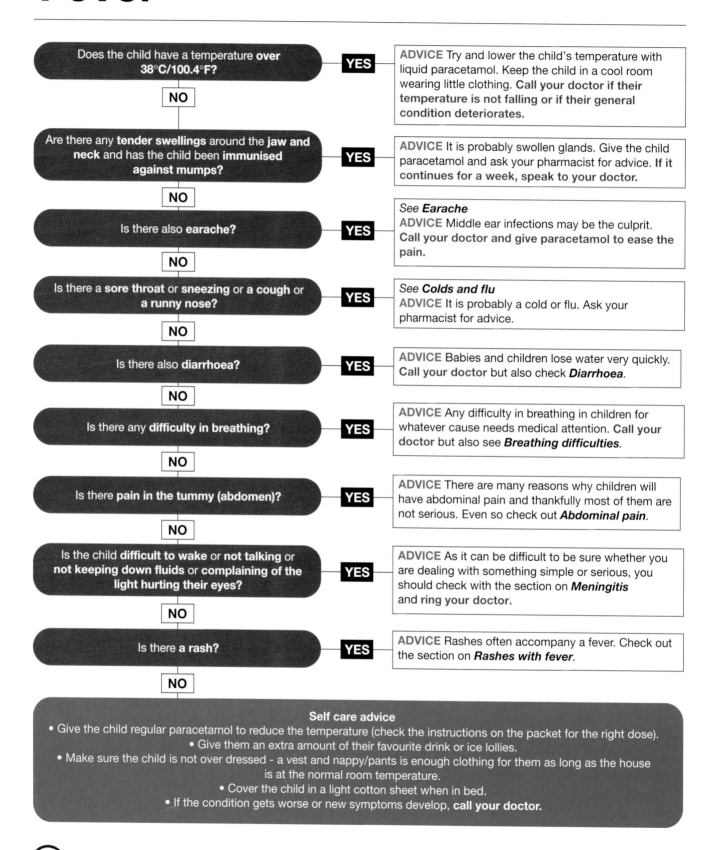

Does the child have a temperature **over 38°C/100.4°F?**

YES — **ADVICE** Try and lower the child's temperature with liquid paracetamol. Keep the child in a cool room wearing little clothing. **Call your doctor if their temperature is not falling or if their general condition deteriorates.**

NO

Are there any **tender swellings** around the **jaw and neck** and has the child been **immunised against mumps?**

YES — **ADVICE** It is probably swollen glands. Give the child paracetamol and ask your pharmacist for advice. If it continues for a week, speak to your doctor.

NO

Is there also **earache?**

YES — *See **Earache*** **ADVICE** Middle ear infections may be the culprit. Call your doctor and give paracetamol to ease the pain.

NO

Is there a **sore throat** or **sneezing** or **a cough** or **a runny nose?**

YES — *See **Colds and flu*** **ADVICE** It is probably a cold or flu. Ask your pharmacist for advice.

NO

Is there also **diarrhoea?**

YES — **ADVICE** Babies and children lose water very quickly. **Call your doctor** but also check ***Diarrhoea.***

NO

Is there any **difficulty in breathing?**

YES — **ADVICE** Any difficulty in breathing in children for whatever cause needs medical attention. **Call your doctor** but also see ***Breathing difficulties.***

NO

Is there **pain in the tummy (abdomen)?**

YES — **ADVICE** There are many reasons why children will have abdominal pain and thankfully most of them are not serious. Even so check out ***Abdominal pain.***

NO

Is the child **difficult to wake** or **not talking** or **not keeping down fluids** or **complaining of the light hurting their eyes?**

YES — **ADVICE** As it can be difficult to be sure whether you are dealing with something simple or serious, you should check with the section on ***Meningitis*** and **ring your doctor.**

NO

Is there **a rash?**

YES — **ADVICE** Rashes often accompany a fever. Check out the section on ***Rashes with fever.***

NO

Self care advice
- Give the child regular paracetamol to reduce the temperature (check the instructions on the packet for the right dose).
- Give them an extra amount of their favourite drink or ice lollies.
- Make sure the child is not over dressed - a vest and nappy/pants is enough clothing for them as long as the house is at the normal room temperature.
- Cover the child in a light cotton sheet when in bed.
- If the condition gets worse or new symptoms develop, **call your doctor.**

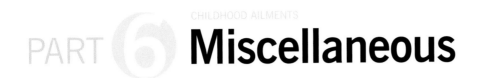

Miscellaneous

Congenital heart disease

Few things worry parents more than congenital defects in their baby's heart. Unfortunately they are not rare, affecting about one baby in 120. Being congenital, they are by definition present from birth, but many not be diagnosed until later on when symptoms such as breathing problems first arise.

It would be easy to get very upset over this issue, but it is worth remembering that most defects will cause no problem to the child and the remainder can often be treated successfully so that they have a normal or near-normal life. Many children will grow into healthy adults without ever realising there is a congenital defect in their heart which has never caused a problem and so was never diagnosed as such. Even the term, 'a hole in the heart' raises the spectre of some sort of gap in the outside wall of the heart rather like a punctured inner tube. Simply understanding the actual way the heart is affected can help reassure.

Congenital heart disease take several forms. The commonest are:
● Openings in the internal wall of the heart ('hole in the heart'). These are called septal defects as the septum separates the two sides of the heart.
● Persistence of a blood channel used only while the baby is in the womb which should close off after birth. This is called patent ductus arteriosus (PDA).
● Narrowing of the main artery of the body, the aorta. This is called aortic stenosis.
● Narrowing of the main heart valves. This is called aortic and pulmonary valve stenosis.
● A complex of all four defects occurring together. This is called Fallot's tetralogy.

All of these defects vary enormously in severity but result in a mixing of oxygenated blood from the lungs with deoxygenated blood returning from the rest of the body. Deoxygenated blood is blue/red in colour while oxygenated blood is bright red. The heart normally keeps them separate, giving the body a pink colour. When they mix, places like the lips especially turn slightly blue, which is made worse when oxygen is in higher demand.

Symptoms

A common symptom is cyanosis, a bluish skin colour especially around the lips, and sufferers are breathless and easily tired. Varying levels of activity can bring this on, along with a characteristic squatting position during recovery. Most murmurs, noises in the heart as blood is being pumped, are innocent but if there is a congenital defect the characteristic murmur can often be heard using a stethoscope.

Causes

Parents often feel guilty, that they somehow brought on the problem in some way. In truth there are many different causes of congenital heart disease:
● Virus infections early in pregnancy, especially German measles (rubella). It is vital that both boys and girls are vaccinated against this infection.
● Some medical drugs, taken in the early weeks of pregnancy. The dreadful Thalidomide tragedy is thankfully very rare. Very few medicines cause harm but all medicines should only be taken under medical advice during pregnancy.
● Some poorly-controlled medical conditions in the mother such as diabetes or Systemic Lupus Erythematosus (SLE). These conditions are treatable during pregnancy and often improve, but more importantly any potential damage to the baby can be minimised by careful monitoring and control.
● Down's syndrome unfortunately may include congenital heart defects, but like the severity of the condition itself, varies enormously between children.

Diagnosis

Generally it is usually the parent who first raises the alarm after seeing a bluish tinge in the skin and breathlessness. Referral to a paediatrician will result in further tests such as a chest X-ray, electrocardiograms (ECG: this picks up electrical activity from the heart), echocardiography (ultrasound to look at how the valves are working) and possibly the passage of fine tubes into the heart (cardiac catheterisation to see where and how the blood is mixing).

Prevention

Most of the problems cannot be prevented other than addressing causes such as uncontrolled medical conditions, avoiding drugs especially during early pregnancy and ensuring immunity from German measles before becoming pregnant.

Complications

Thankfully, modern surgery reduces the complications to a minimum but otherwise there can be poor growth, thickening (clubbing) of the tips of the fingers and toes, poor ability to remain active, chest and possibly other infections and a danger of the heart itself being infected.

Treatment

Surgical correction of the congenital defect is often advised during infancy or childhood. Often this will involve two stages, the last being performed when the child is older. All children will benefit from treatment and most will have normal or near-normal lives so it is important to alert your doctor or health visitor to any problems such as breathlessness or blue colouration of the lips.

Febrile convulsions

Febrile convulsions are quite common in young children, but the great majority of children who suffer these episodes are not epileptic and these fits do not occur because of any brain defect, nor do they mean that the child will develop epilepsy in future. High body temperature is invariably the cause.

Around 3 or 4 children out of 1000 will have a febrile convulsion by the time they are five years old. In most cases the fits occur after the age of six months; they typically occur between the ages of 6 months and 6 years.

Symptoms
Febrile convulsions seldom last for longer than a few minutes, and although the child may take a few minutes to recover, their final recovery is complete.

Causes
Conditions commonly causing fevers include middle ear infection (otitis media), tonsillitis, kidney or urinary infection, pneumonia and any of the common infectious diseases of childhood such as measles, mumps, chicken pox and whooping cough. Even the common cold or flu can be a trigger.

Any illness causing a temperature higher than 39°C (102.2°F) can set off a febrile convulsion.

Diagnosis
If the convulsions cease when the child's temperature drops this gives an obvious diagnosis, but they should still be reported to your doctor.

Prevention
High temperatures can be brought down with simple things like cooling the room, removing clothing and tepid sponging (using a flannel or sponge to apply tepid water which then evaporates, cooling the child). Medicines such as paediatric ibuprofen, paracetamol liquid medicine or paracetamol suppositories (tablets that you place inside the child's bottom) will also help. Any seizure for whatever cause should be reported to your doctor, although you may not always need a visit.

Complications
Injury from hitting hard objects is a possibility and prolonged seizures due to high temperature can cause brain damage.

Umbilical hernia

There are often things that can happen to a baby which appear serious but which are common, sort themselves out or can be treated very easily. Umbilical hernias are a good example.

Symptoms
A bulge is seen or felt close to the belly button which is soft but not painful. It can often disappear on its own only to return a few days later.

Causes
For a while after being born, the muscle layer around the belly button (umbilicus) can be weak or even have a small gap in it. Not surprisingly, some of the inside of the abdomen can protrude through causing a 'hernia'. This can range from a small amount of fatty tissue to part of the intestine itself. Umbilical hernias are most likely to appear in the first three weeks of life as your baby's belly button heals up after the birth and they are twice as common in boys as in girls. Anything which increases the pressure inside the abdomen such as crying, laughing, or coughing can make the hernia appear larger.

Treatment
Fortunately the majority of umbilical hernias correct themselves by two to three years old but occasionally surgery is needed after this age to strengthen the area around the tummy button and hold in the bulge. Most doctors prefer to wait and see if the hernia gets larger after the first year or resolves itself. Generally, doctors will only recommend surgery if the hernia hasn't gone away by three years old or progressively worsens in the first few years.

Self care
It is worth keeping an eye on any bulge around your baby's umbilical cord stump (newborns) or tummy button (older babies and toddlers). If it feels hot, changes colour (especially blue) or is tender you must phone your doctor. If the child is passing blood in their motions or vomiting repeatedly you must call 999/112.

The hernia should be disappearing by the age of 2, so if it is still there ask your doctor's advice.

Shock (loss of blood)

Children in shock may become pale, sweaty, drowsy and confused. They need urgent medical attention. While waiting for help, remain calm but do not give them anything to eat or drink. If they are unconscious lie them on their back with their legs raised, loosen any tight clothing and keep them warm.

Crying baby

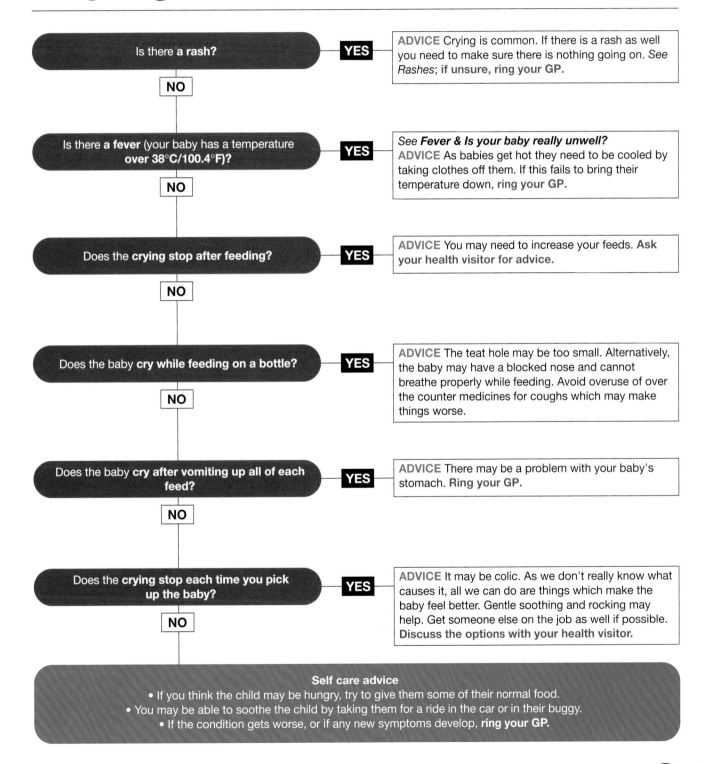

Is there a rash? — **YES** → **ADVICE** Crying is common. If there is a rash as well you need to make sure there is nothing going on. *See Rashes*; **if unsure, ring your GP.**

NO

Is there a fever (your baby has a temperature over 38°C/100.4°F)? — **YES** → *See **Fever & Is your baby really unwell?*** **ADVICE** As babies get hot they need to be cooled by taking clothes off them. If this fails to bring their temperature down, **ring your GP.**

NO

Does the crying stop after feeding? — **YES** → **ADVICE** You may need to increase your feeds. **Ask your health visitor for advice.**

NO

Does the baby cry while feeding on a bottle? — **YES** → **ADVICE** The teat hole may be too small. Alternatively, the baby may have a blocked nose and cannot breathe properly while feeding. Avoid overuse of over the counter medicines for coughs which may make things worse.

NO

Does the baby cry after vomiting up all of each feed? — **YES** → **ADVICE** There may be a problem with your baby's stomach. **Ring your GP.**

NO

Does the crying stop each time you pick up the baby? — **YES** → **ADVICE** It may be colic. As we don't really know what causes it, all we can do are things which make the baby feel better. Gentle soothing and rocking may help. Get someone else on the job as well if possible. **Discuss the options with your health visitor.**

NO

Self care advice
- If you think the child may be hungry, try to give them some of their normal food.
- You may be able to soothe the child by taking them for a ride in the car or in their buggy.
- If the condition gets worse, or if any new symptoms develop, **ring your GP.**

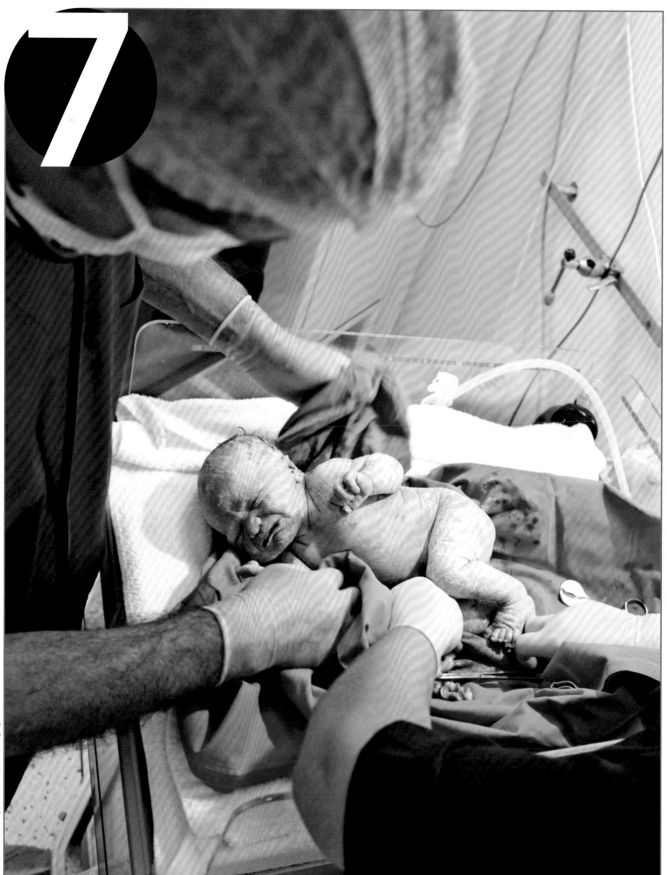

PART **7** **Reference**

The Apgar score

The score is normally taken 1 minute after birth and again after 5 minutes.

A score of 7 or more (out of a possible 10) is good. A score between 4 and 7 may mean that some extra help with breathing is needed. A score below 4 calls for immediate resuscitation.

Note that there are many possible reasons for a low Apgar score. Provided effective action is taken, a low score does not necessarily indicate future problems. Likewise, an initial score of 10 is virtually unknown.

Sign	Score 0	Score 1	Score 2
Appearance (colour)	Blue or pale all over	Pink body, blue hands and feet	Pink all over
Pulse rate	No pulse	Below 100 per minute	Above 100 per minute
Grimace (reflex irritability)	No response	Grimace	Vigorous cry
Activity	Weak and floppy	Some movement	Very active
Respiration	Not breathing	Slow and/or irregular	Good breathing

Service Record

Some time in the years ahead, your son or daughter is going to ask 'Dad, when did I cut my first tooth/say my first words/learn to use a potty?' Or you may find that your own recollection of when something happened is at variance with your partner's. If you are still at the stage when lack of sleep means that your memory is no longer entirely reliable, these pages will be invaluable.

Birth

Baby's name. . . . .

Date and time of birth. . . . .

Place of birth . . . .

Type of birth . . . .

Birth weight . . . .

Date of leaving hospital . . . .

Other notes. . . . .

. . . .

. . . .

What's that in old money?

Metrication notwithstanding, older relatives may want to know the baby's weight in pounds and ounces. Here's a chart:

To convert exactly, multiply the weight in kilograms by 2.205 to get the weight in pounds, then multiply the decimal part of the weight in pounds by 16 to get the ounces.

So for example:
2.850 kilograms x 2.205 = 6.28425 lb
0.28425 lb x 16 = 4.548 oz
Weight to nearest whole ounce = 6 lb 5 oz.

kilograms	pounds and ounces (to nearest whole ounce)
2.4	5 lb 5 oz
2.5	5 lb 8 oz
2.6	5 lb 12 oz
2.7	5 lb 15 oz
2.8	6 lb 3 oz
2.9	6 lb 6 oz
3.0	6 lb 10 oz
3.1	6 lb 13 oz
3.2	7 lb 1 oz
3.3	7 lb 4 oz
3.4	7 lb 8 oz
3.5	7 lb 12 oz
3.6	7 lb 15 oz
3.7	8 lb 3 oz
3.8	8 lb 6 oz
3.9	8 lb 10 oz
4.0	8 lb 13 oz

Development

First smile. . . . .

First laugh. . . . .

First unbroken night's sleep . . . .

First tooth . . . .

Starts solid foods . . . .

Weaned . . . .

Sits up . . . .

Learns to crawl . . . .

Stands with support. . . . .

Stands unaided . . . .

First steps . . . .

First words . . . .

Knows own name . . . .

Climbs stairs . . . .

Potty trained . . . .

Medical records

Illnesses . . . .

Allergies . . . .

Accidents . . . .

Other problems . . . .

. . . .

Immunisations

Triple vaccine (diphtheria, tetanus, pertussis) . . . .

Hib . . . .

Meningococcal type C . . . .

Polio . . . .

BCG (tuberculosis) (if applicable) . . . .

Measles, mumps and rubella (MMR) . . . .

Diptheria, tetanus and polio booster . . . .

MMR booster . . . .

Others . . . .

. . . .

Contact details

GP . . . .

Health visitor. . . . .

Hospital . . . .

Dentist . . . .

Nursery or playgroup . . . .

Childminder . . . .

Babysitter . . . .

Others . . . .

. . . .

. . . .

Dimensions and weights

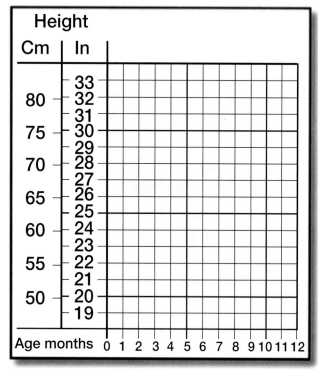

Height

Cm	In
80	33 / 32 / 31
75	30
70	29 / 28 / 27
65	26 / 25
60	24 / 23
55	22 / 21
50	20 / 19

Age months 0 1 2 3 4 5 6 7 8 9 10 11 12

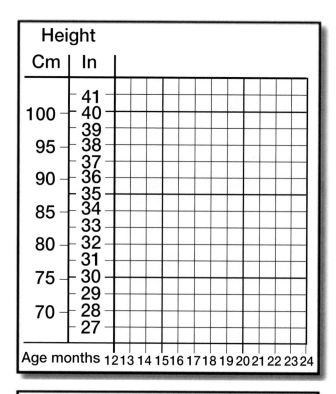

Height

Cm	In
100	41 / 40 / 39
95	38 / 37
90	36 / 35
85	34 / 33
80	32 / 31
75	30 / 29
70	28 / 27

Age months 12 13 14 15 16 17 18 19 20 21 22 23 24

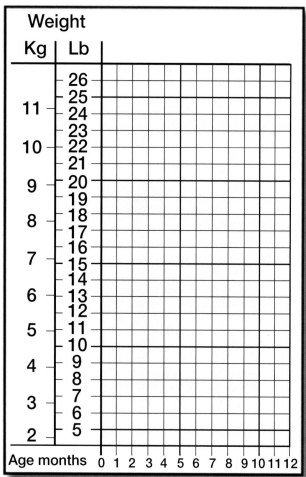

Weight

Kg	Lb
11	26 / 25 / 24 / 23 / 22 / 21
10	20 / 19
9	18 / 17
8	16 / 15
7	14
6	13 / 12 / 11
5	10
4	9 / 8 / 7
3	6
2	5

Age months 0 1 2 3 4 5 6 7 8 9 10 11 12

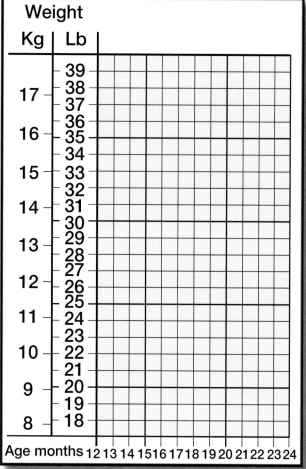

Weight

Kg	Lb
17	39 / 38 / 37 / 36
16	35 / 34
15	33 / 32
14	31 / 30
13	29 / 28 / 27
12	26 / 25
11	24 / 23
10	22 / 21
9	20 / 19
8	18

Age months 12 13 14 15 16 17 18 19 20 21 22 23 24

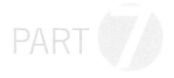

Contacts

Alcoholics anonymous
Tel 0845 769 7555
www.alcoholics-anonymous.org.uk

Breastfeeding line
Tel 0870 444 8708
9am-6pm

British Infertility Counsellors Association
www.bica.net

The British Red Cross
Tel 0870 170 7000
www.redcross.org.uk

Community Hygiene Concern
Tel 020 7686 4321
www.chc.org

Cot Death helpline (The Foundation for the Study of Infant Deaths)
Tel 020 7233 2090
Mon-Fri 9am-11pm, Sat-Sun 6pm-11pm
www.sids.org.uk

Donor Conception Network
Tel 0208 245 4369
www.dcnetwork.org

Drinkline
Tel 0800 917 8282
www.patient.co.uk
www.wrecked.co.uk

Epilepsy Action
0808 800 5050
www.epilepsy.org.uk

Family Planning Association
Tel 0845 122 8690
Mon-Fri 9am-6pm
www.fpa.org.uk

Human Fertilisation and Embryology Authority (HFEA)
Tel 020 7291 8200
Mon-Fri 9am-5pm
www.hfea.gov.uk

The Infertility Network UK
Tel 8701 188 088
www.infertilitynetworkuk.com

Inland Revenue
www.hmrc.gov.uk

The Meningitis Research Foundation
Tel 080 8800 334
www.meningitis.org

The Meningitis Trust
Tel 0800 028 18 28
www.meningitis-trust.org

Miscarriage Association
Tel 01924 200 799
Mon-Fri 9am-4pm
www.miscarriageassociation.org.uk

National Childbirth Trust
Tel 0870 444 8707
Mon-Thurs 9am-5pm, Fri 9am-4pm
www.nct.org.uk

NHS Direct
Tel 0845 46 47
www.nhsdirect.nhs.uk

Pregnancy and birth line
Tel 0870 444 8709
Mon-Fri 10am-8pm

The Prevention and Treatment of Head Lice
Tel 020 7210 4850
9am-5pm
www.dh.gov.uk

Quitline
Tel 0800 00 22 00
www.quit.org.uk

Raising kids
Tel 0208 444 4852
www.raisingkids.co.uk

Relate
www.relate.org.uk

The Sexual Dysfunction Association
Tel 0870 774 3571
www.sda.net

Sexual Health Direct (Run by the Family Planning Association)
Tel 0845 122 8690
Mon-Fri 9am-6pm
www.fpa.org.uk

St John Ambulance
Tel 08700 10 49 50
www.st-john-ambulance.org.uk

Working Families
Tel 0800 013 0313
www.workingfamilies.org.uk

Credits

Babies	Augusta Haynes, Anna Hughes and Sofia Tanswell
Cover design	Pete Shoemark
Editor	Ian Barnes
Editorial director	Matthew Minter
Hints and tips	Hilary Adams, Ruth Allen, Denise Barthorpe, Rob Betts, Mary-Rose Clark, J and Valencia Haynes, Mark Hughes, Carol Limer, Jayne Millet, Matthew Minter, Valerie Moore, Emma Parsons, Nicola Poulton, Steve Rendle, Alison Roelich, Pete Shoemark, Rachael Smith, Carole Turk, Karen Wallace, Kirsty Waterton, Bow Watkinson and Em Willmott
Loan of doll	Martha Minter
Model for baby carrier	Mark Hughes
Page build	James Robertson
Photography	All photos are from istockphoto.com, except Paul Tanswell (pages 91, 95, 98, 99, 101 and 139) J Haynes (cover and page 113) and Tracey Robertson (page 34).
Production control	Charles Seaton
Technical illustrations	Mark Stevens, Matthew Marke and Roger Healing